I0503777

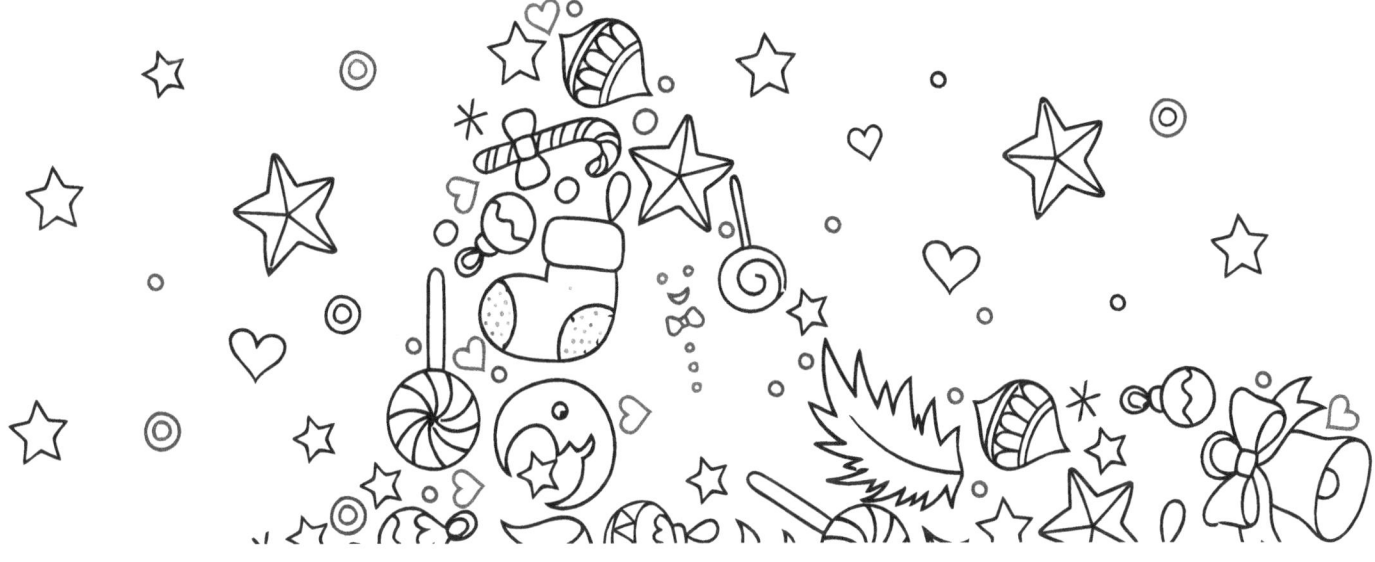

This Christmas Coloring Book
Belongs To:

_____

_____

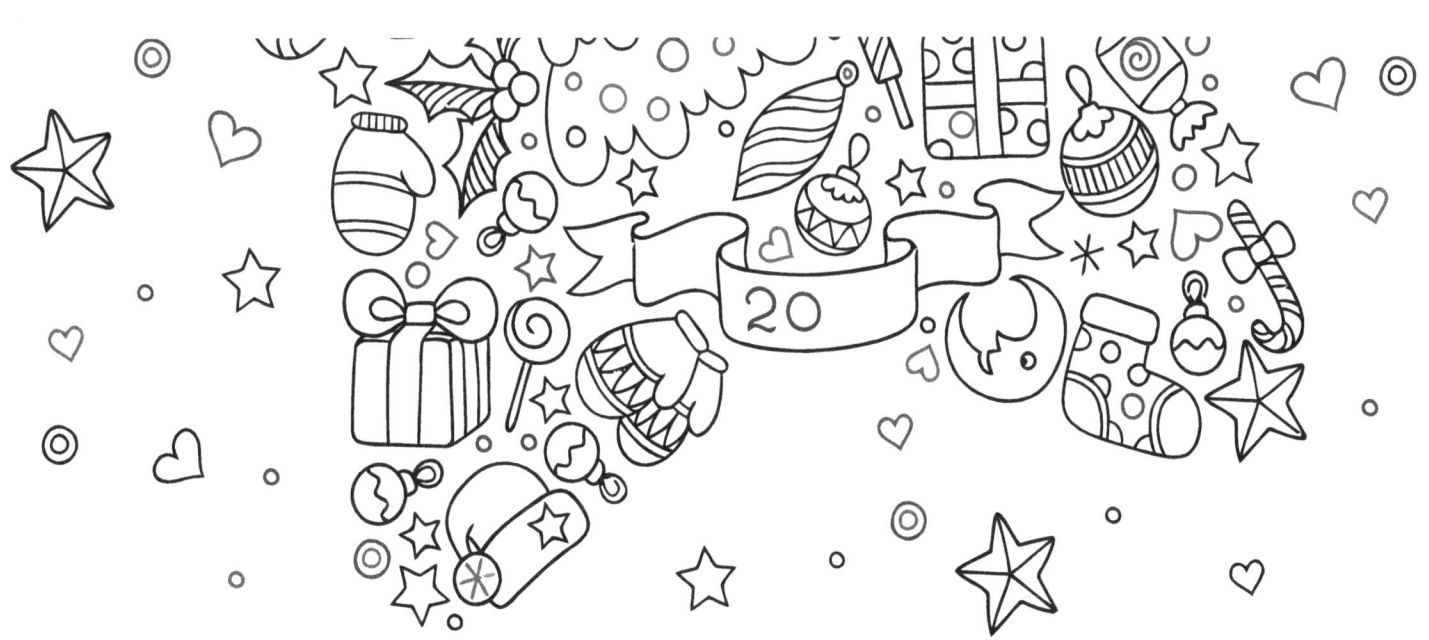

Write and Draw to Express Yourself

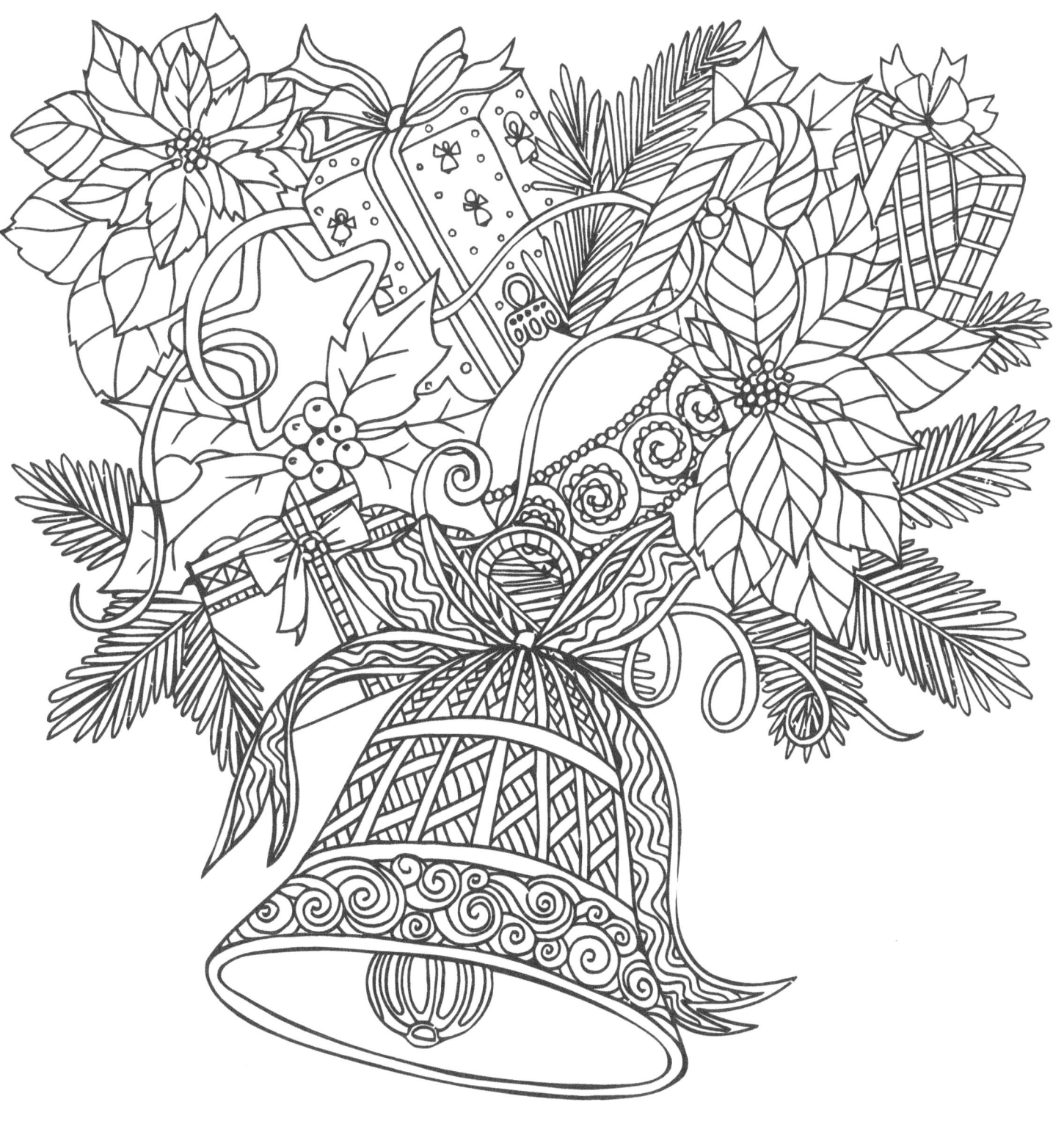

Write and Draw to Express Yourself

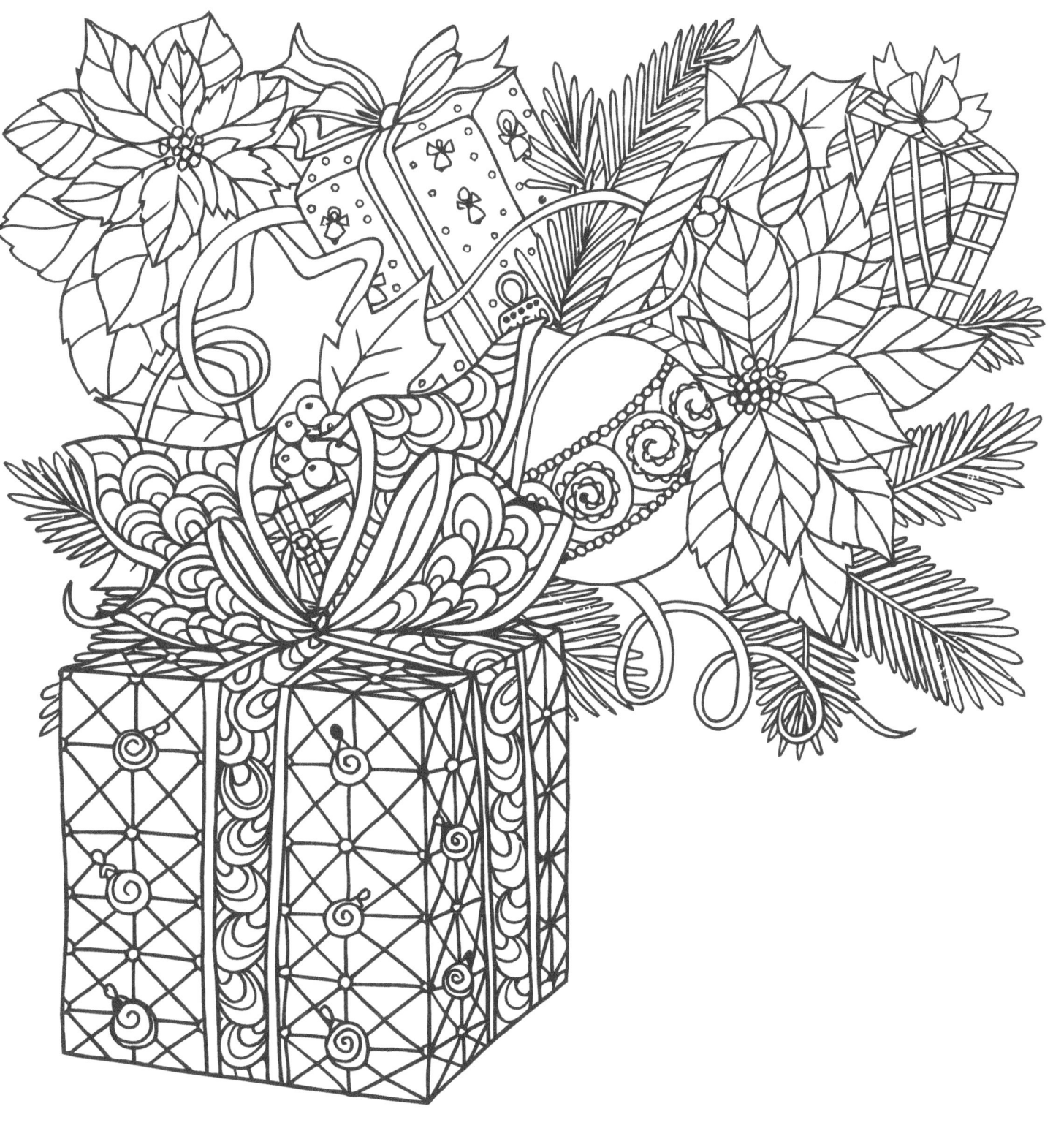

Write and Draw to Express Yourself

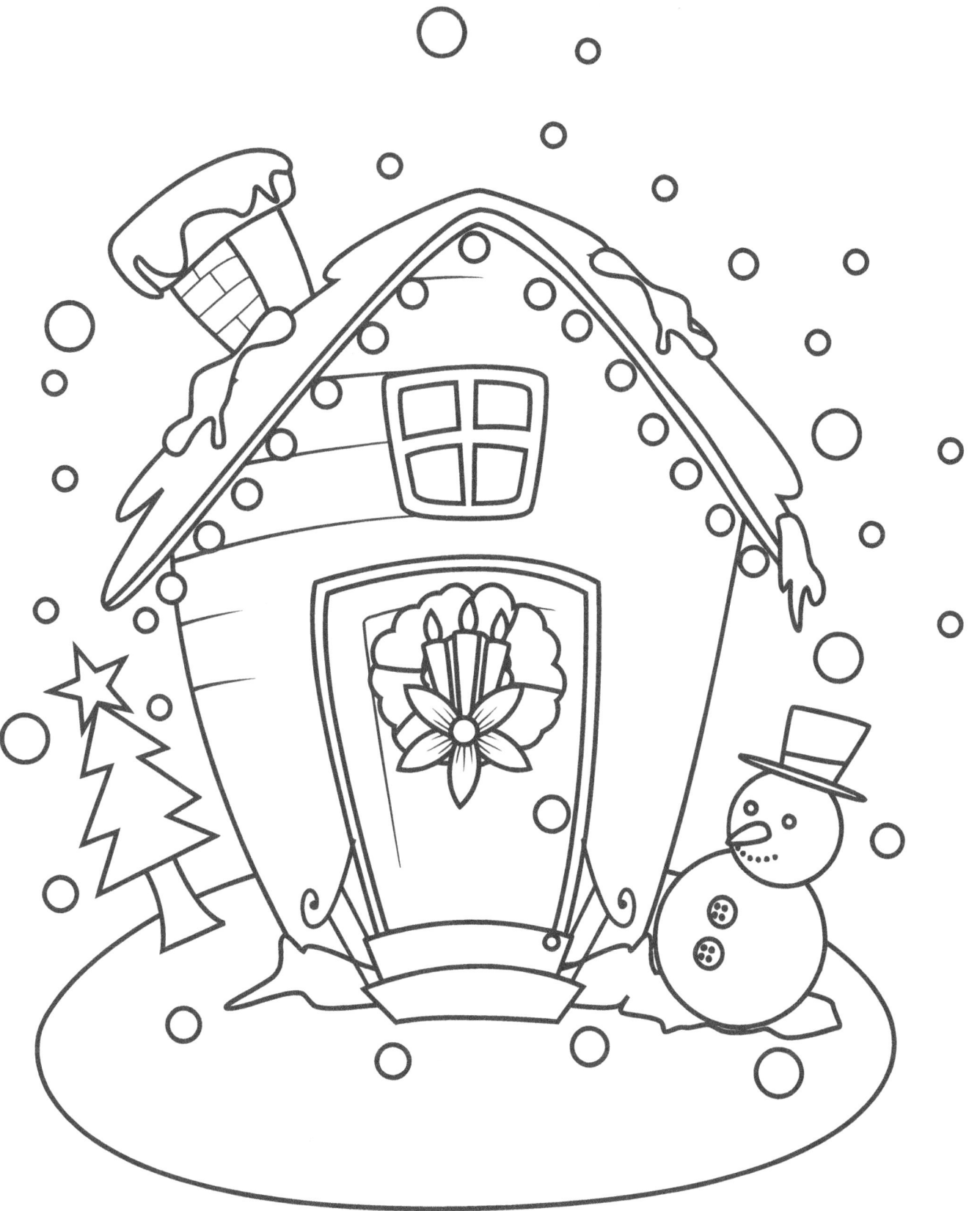

Write and Draw to Express Yourself

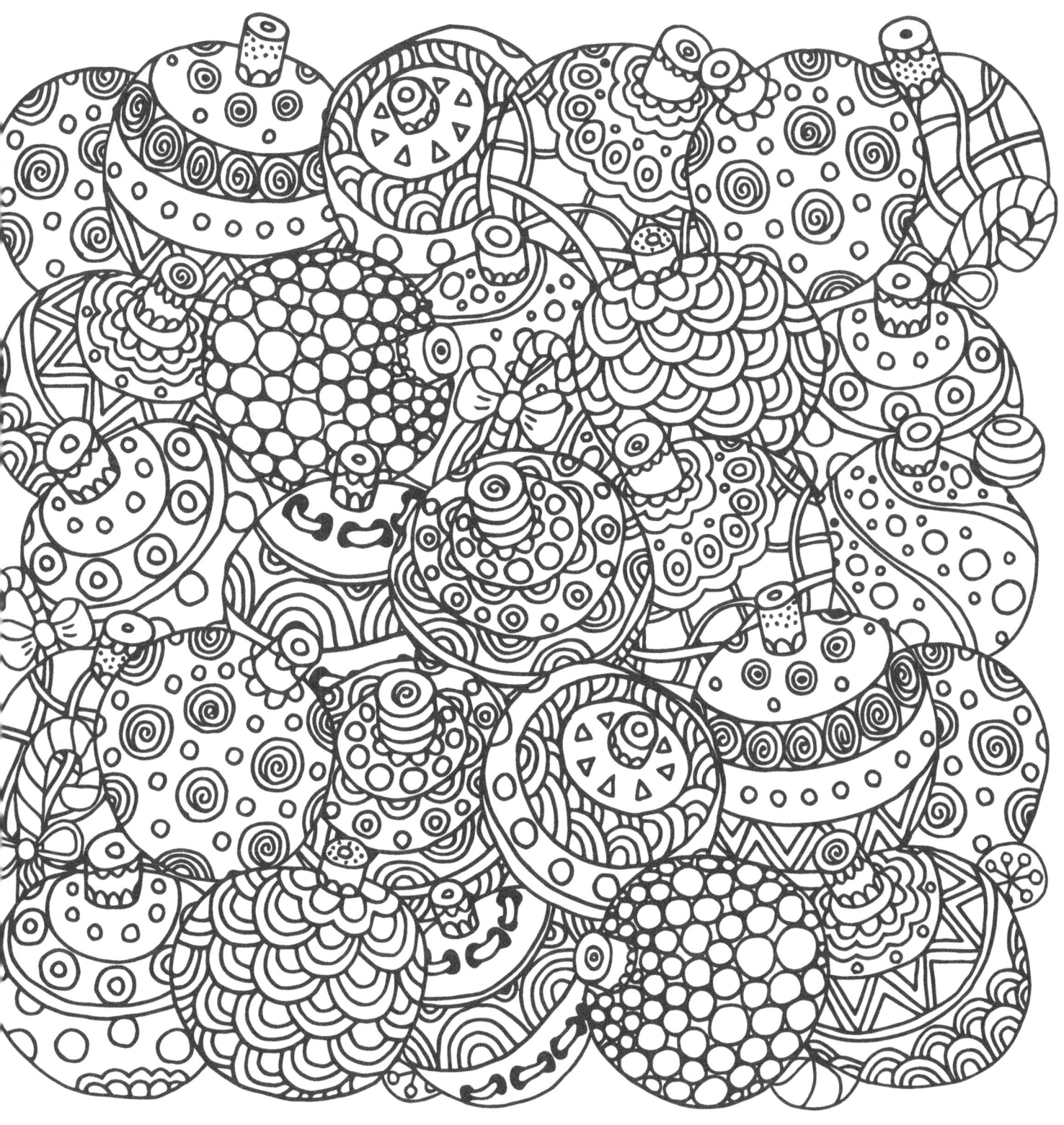

Write and Draw to Express Yourself

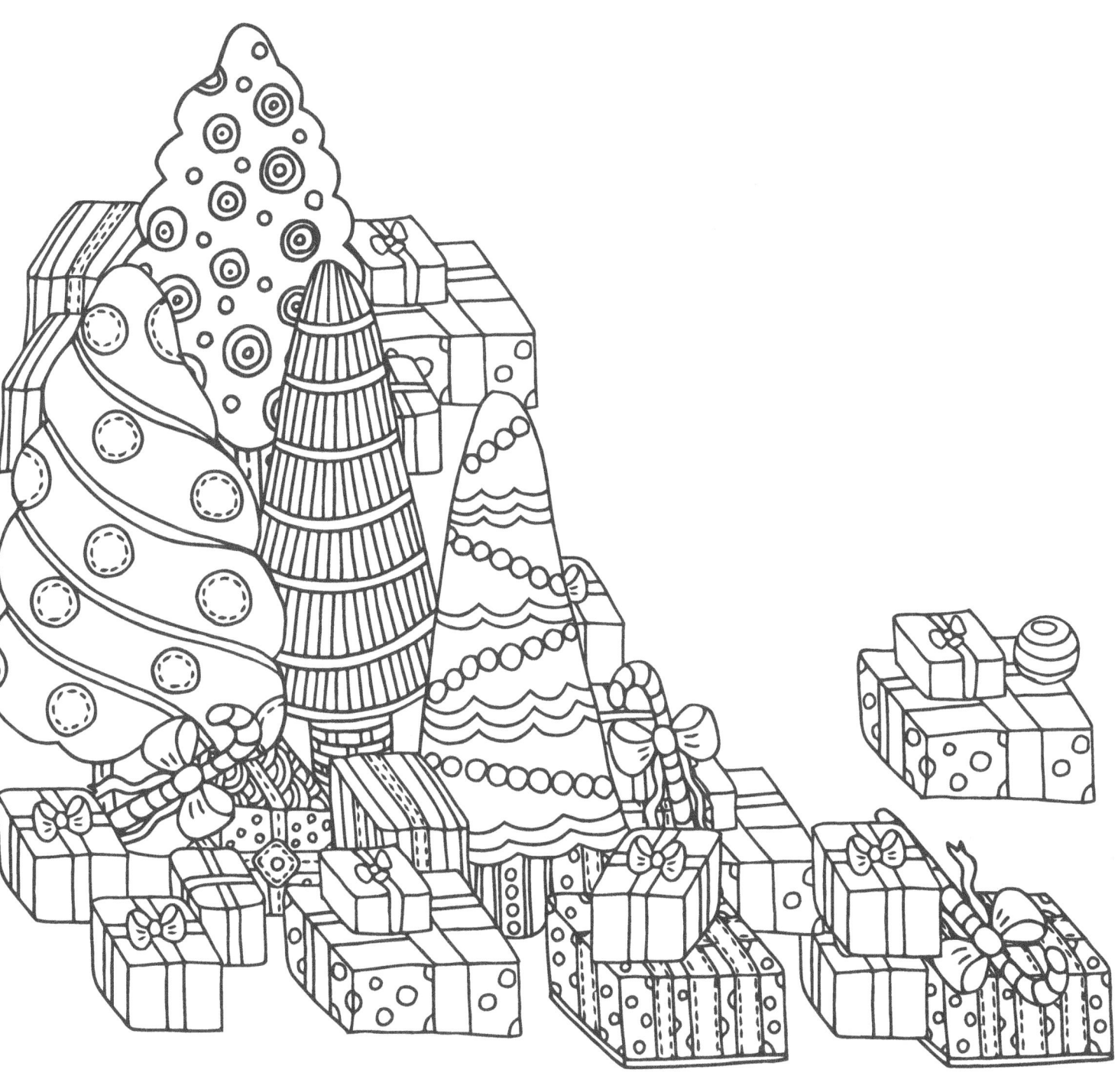

Write and Draw to Express Yourself

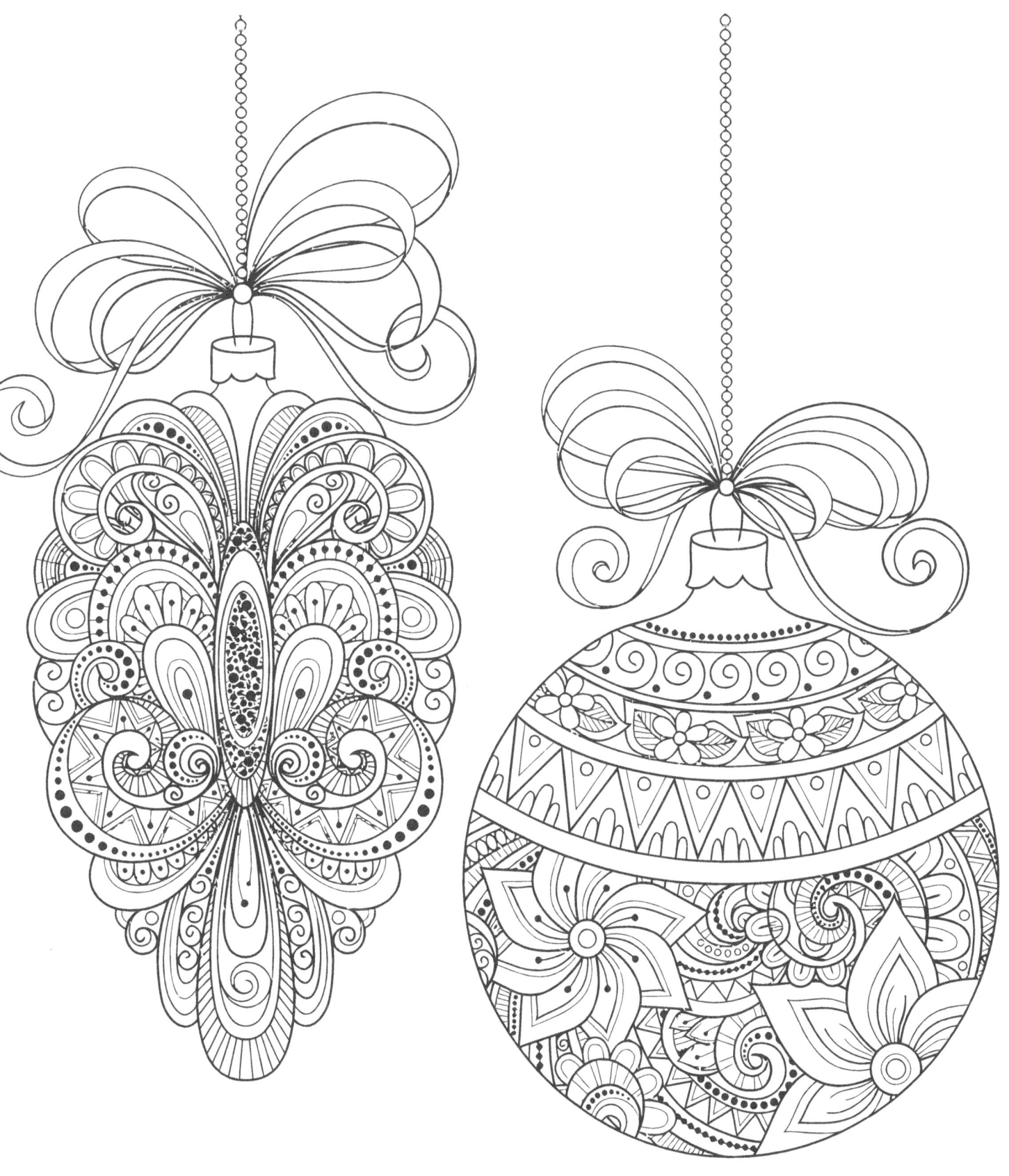

Date: _____/_____/_____

Write and Draw to Express Yourself

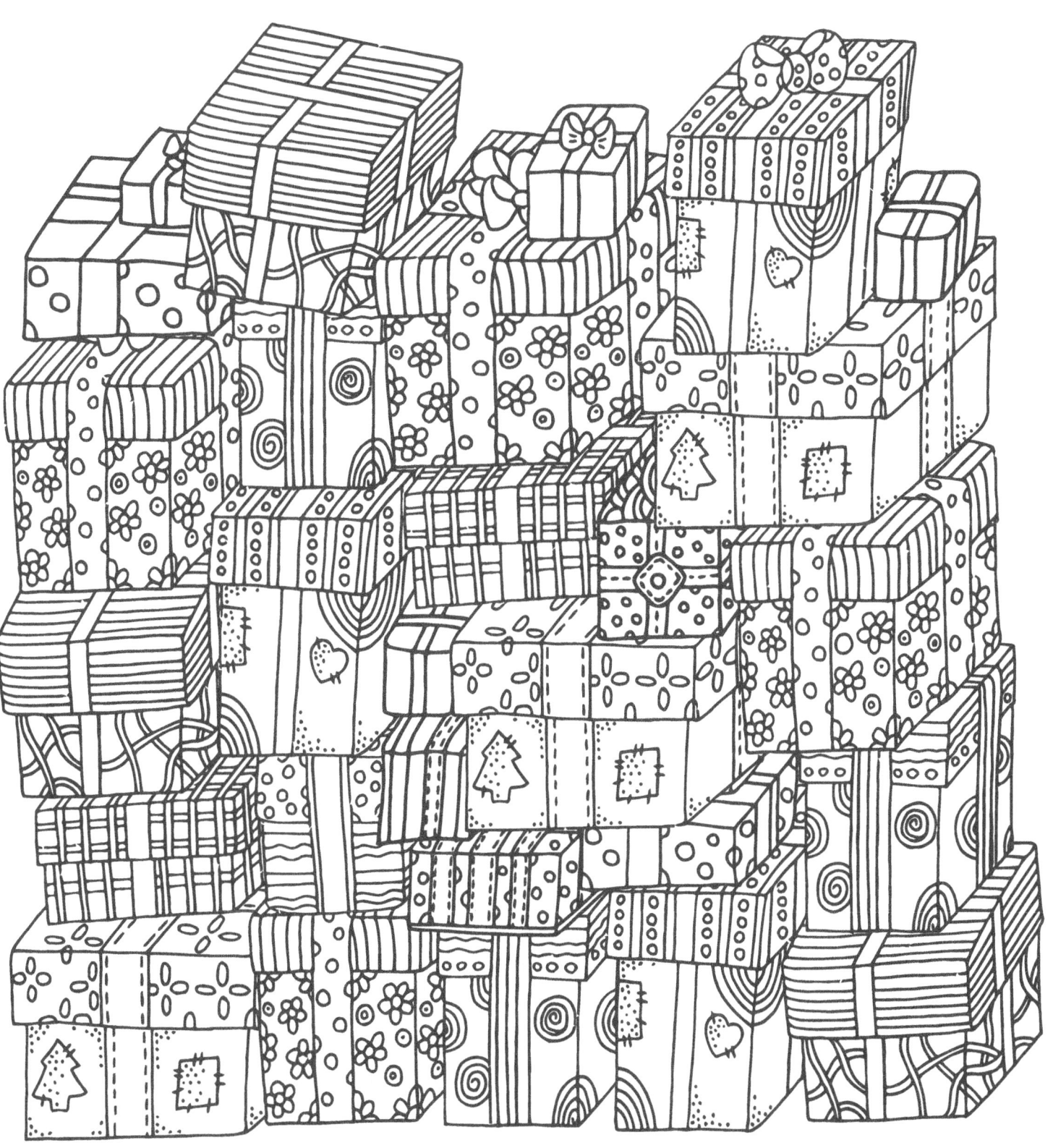

Write and Draw to Express Yourself

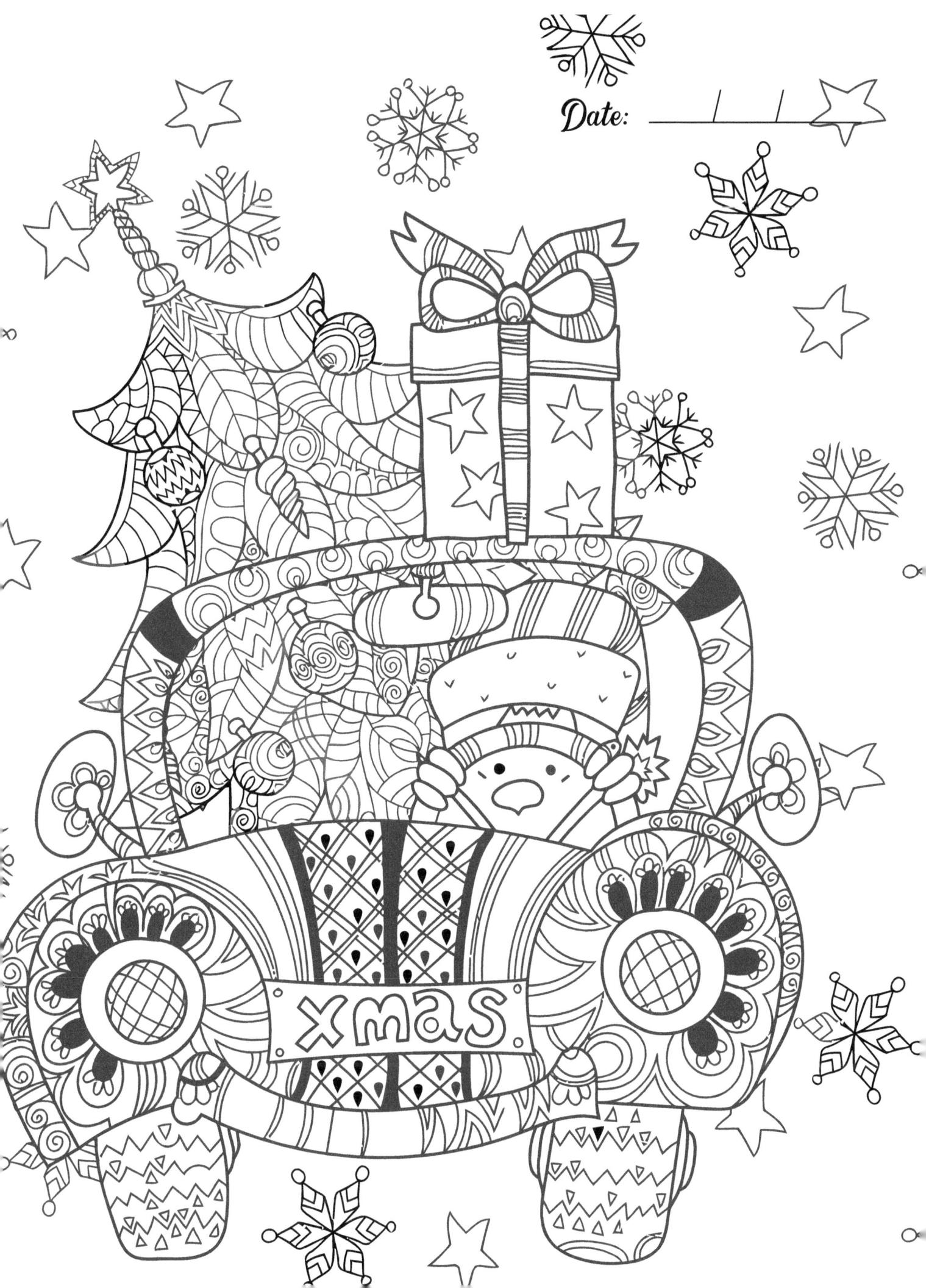

Date: ___/___/___

Write and Draw to Express Yourself

Date:

Write and Draw to Express Yourself

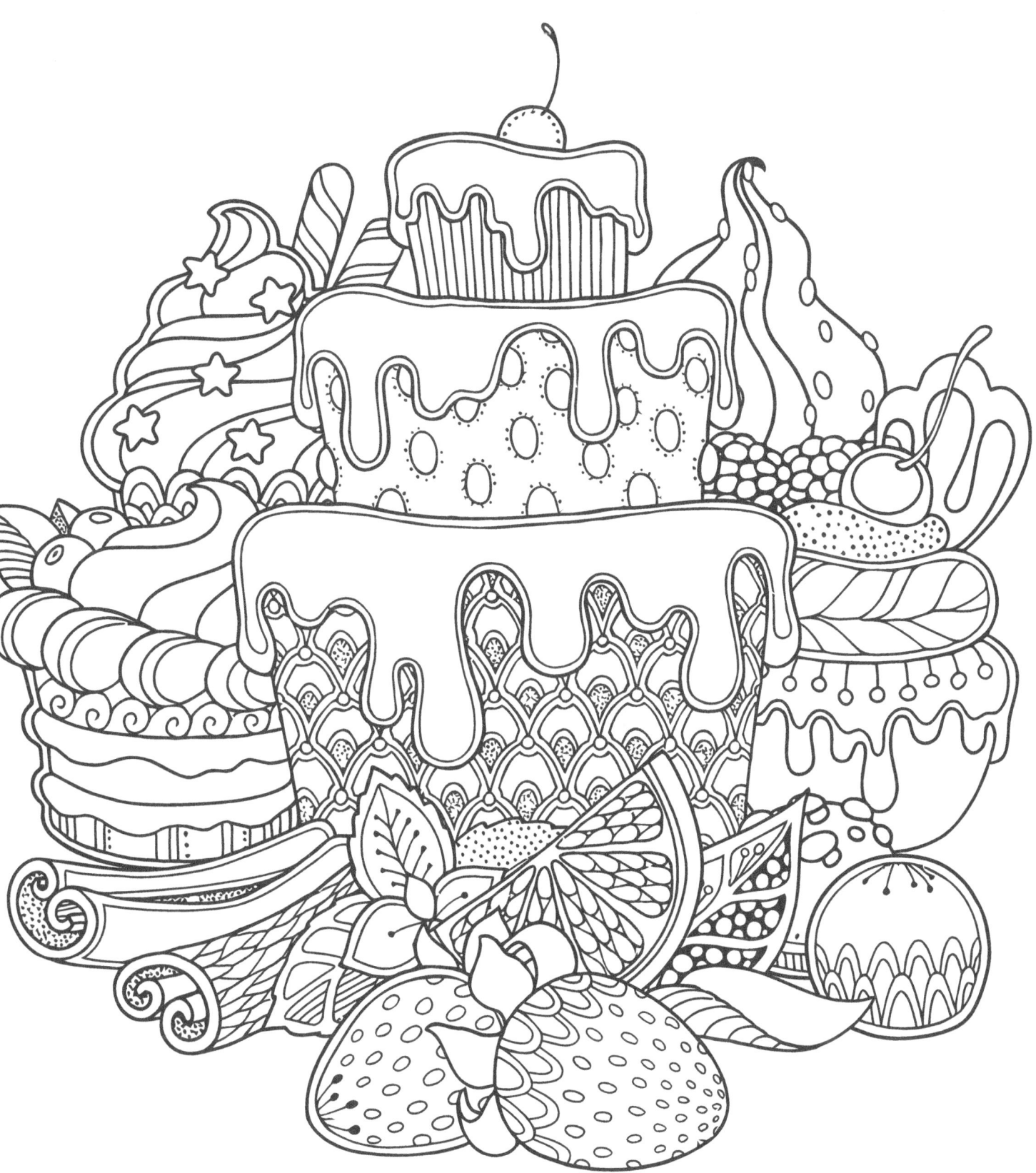

Write and Draw to Express Yourself

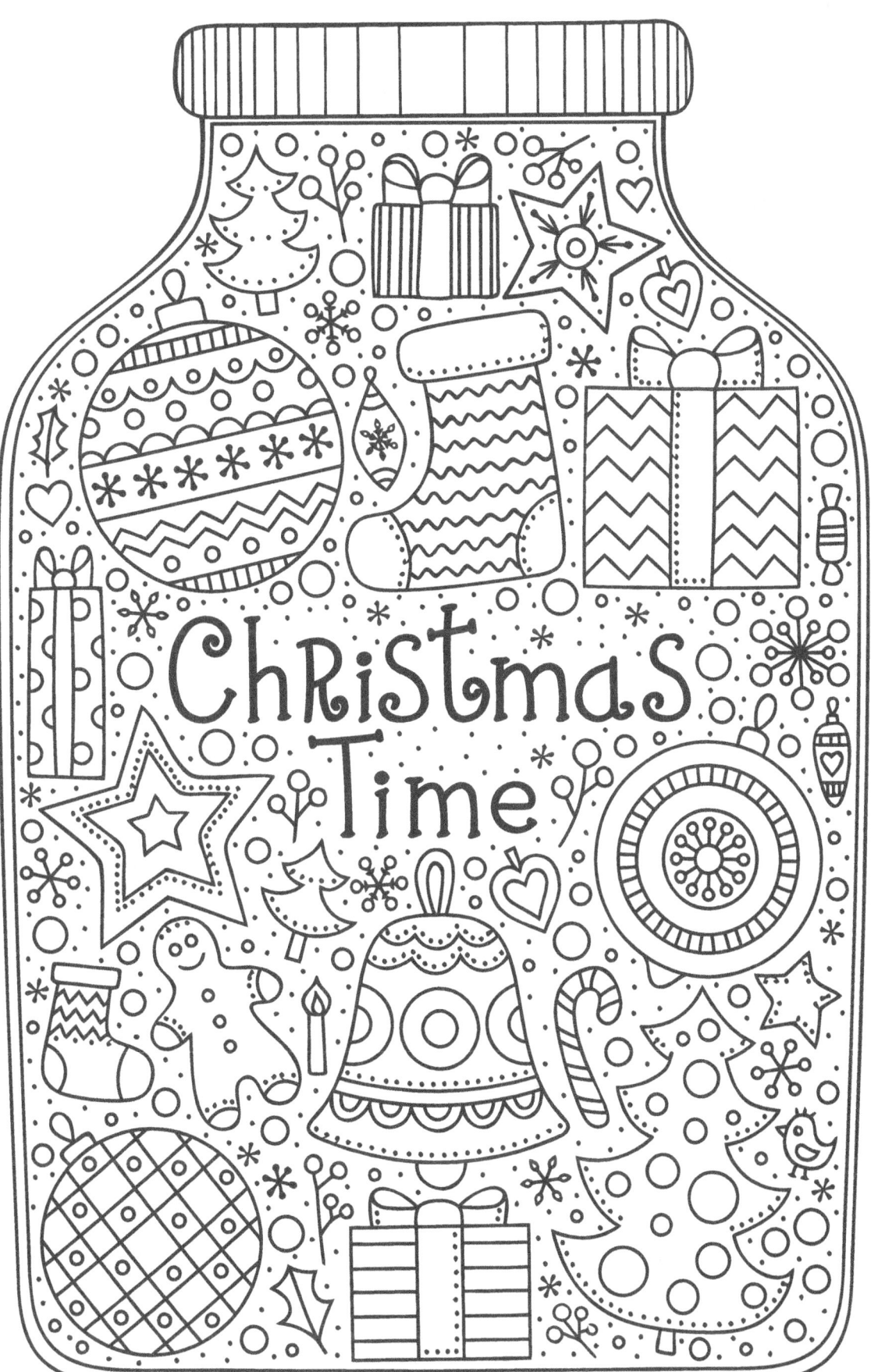

Write and Draw to Express Yourself

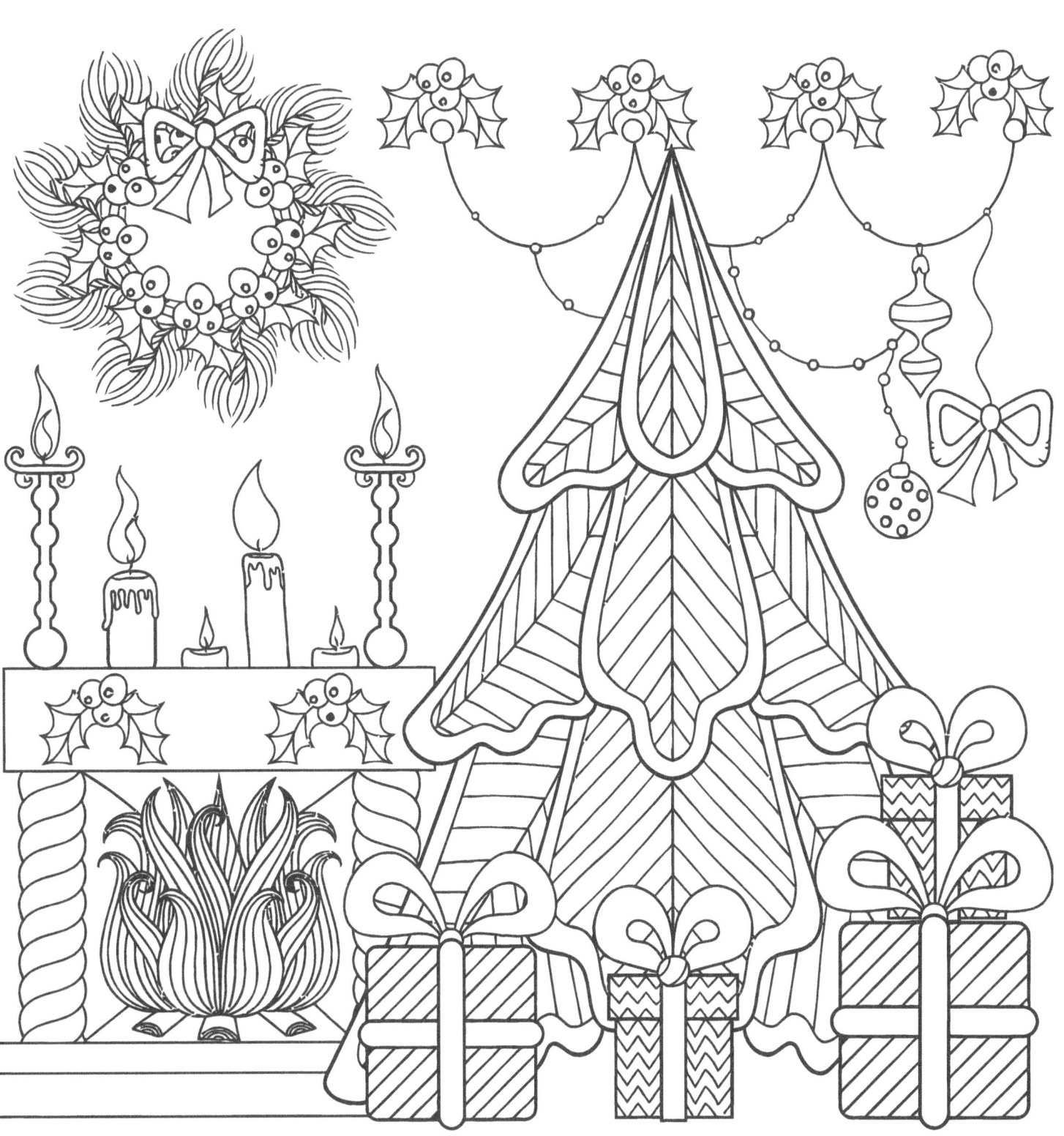

Write and Draw to Express Yourself

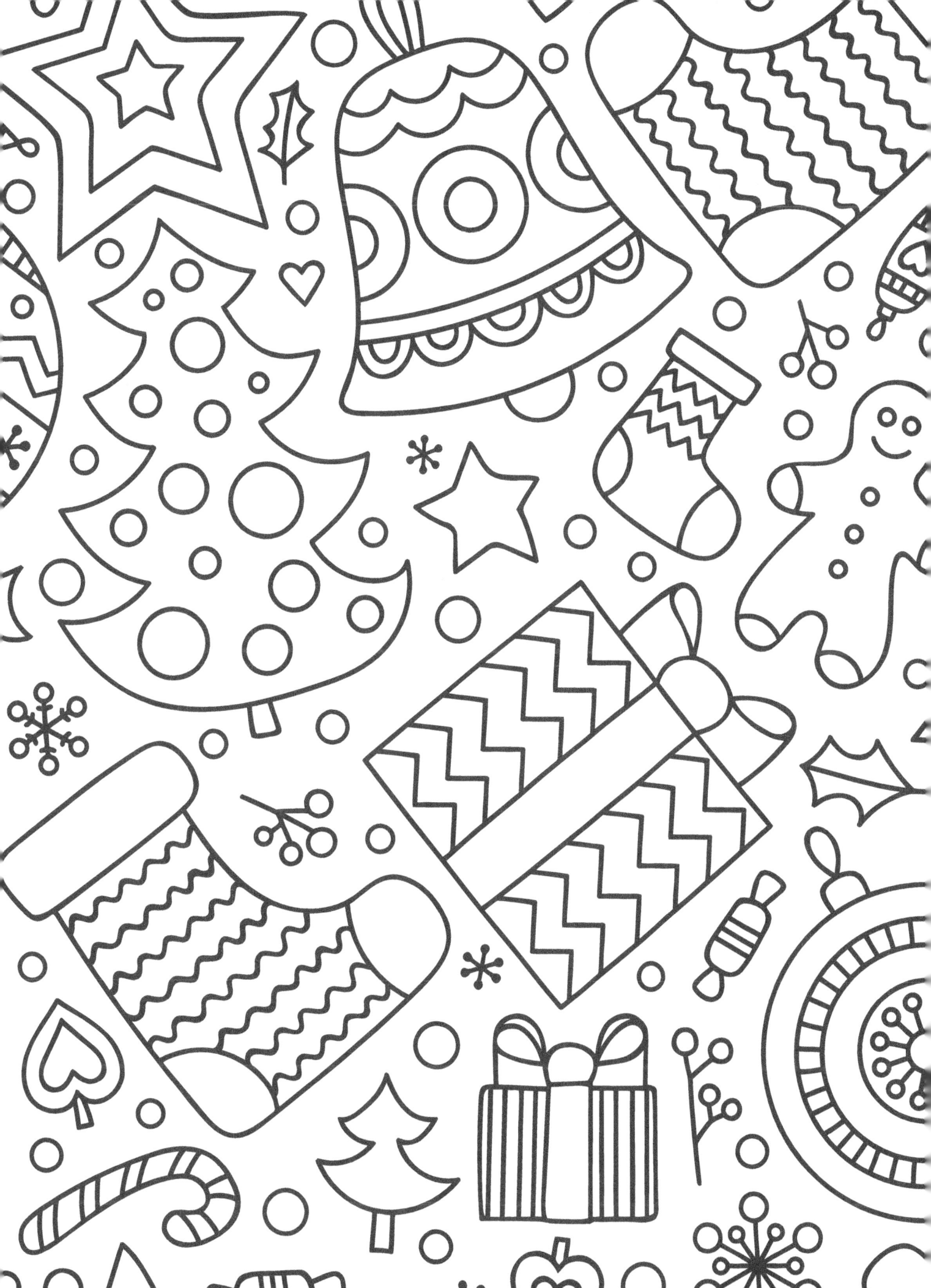

Write and Draw to Express Yourself

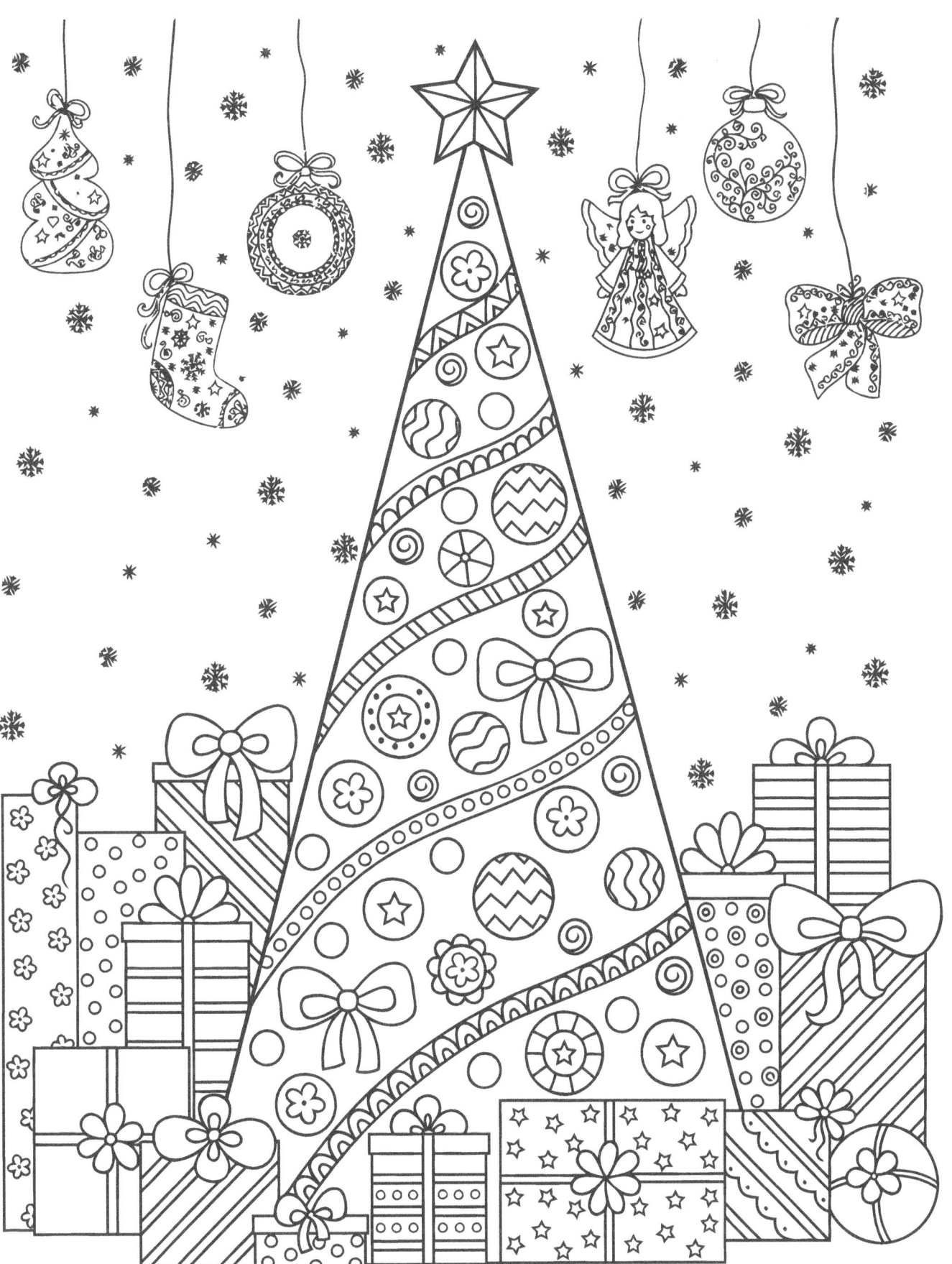

Write and Draw to Express Yourself

Write and Draw to Express Yourself

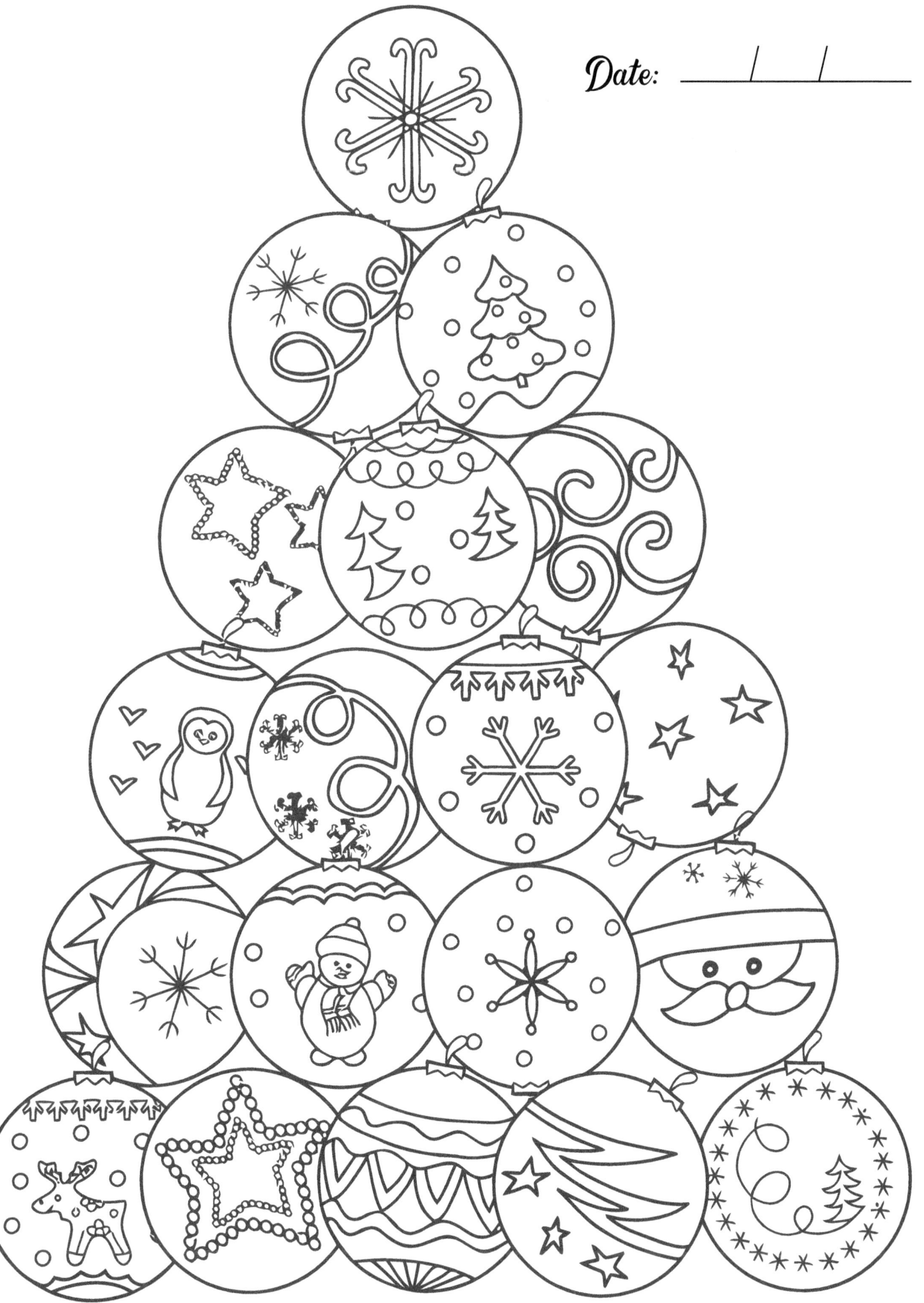

Date: _____ / ____ / _____

Write and Draw to Express Yourself

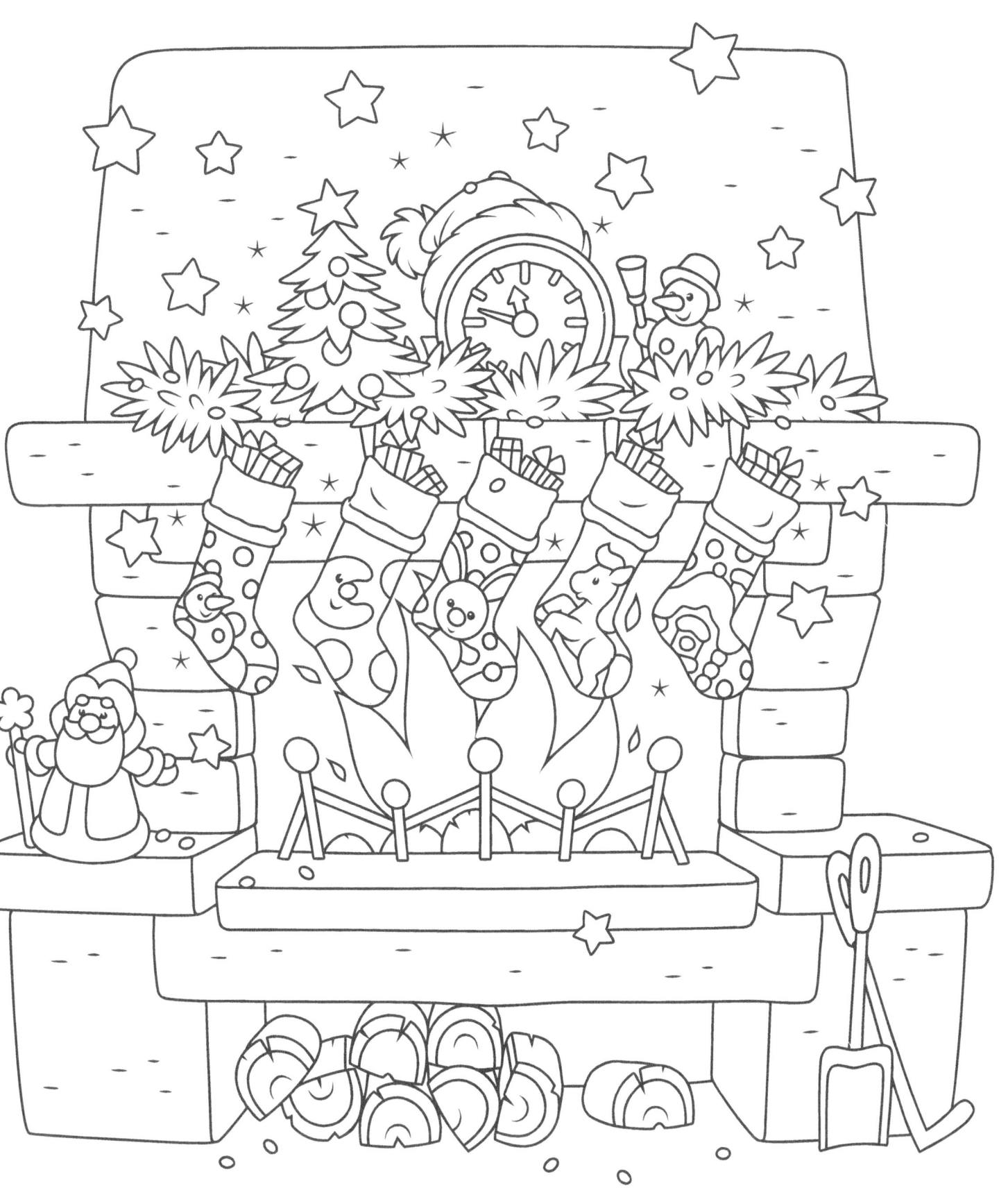

Write and Draw to Express Yourself

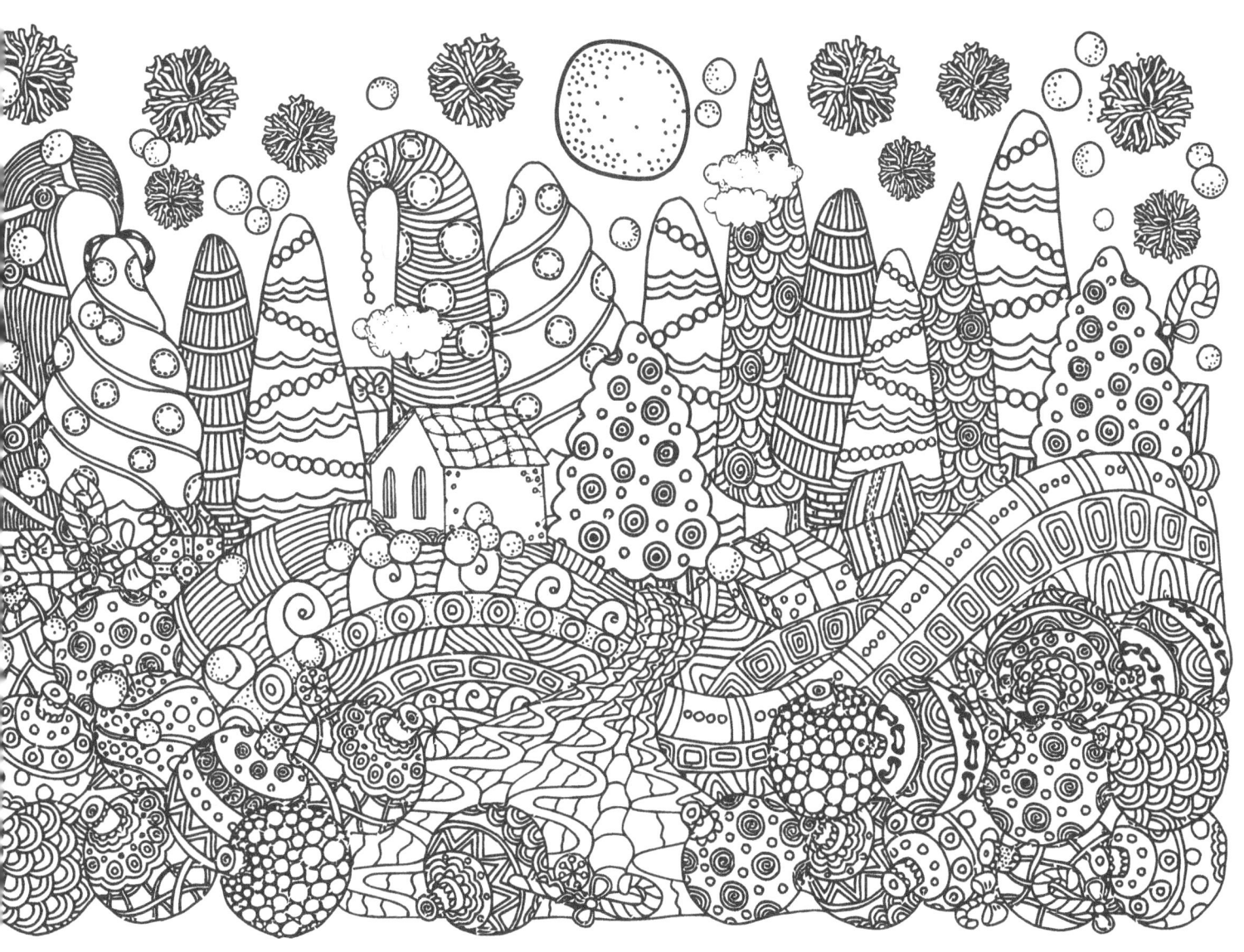

Write and Draw to Express Yourself

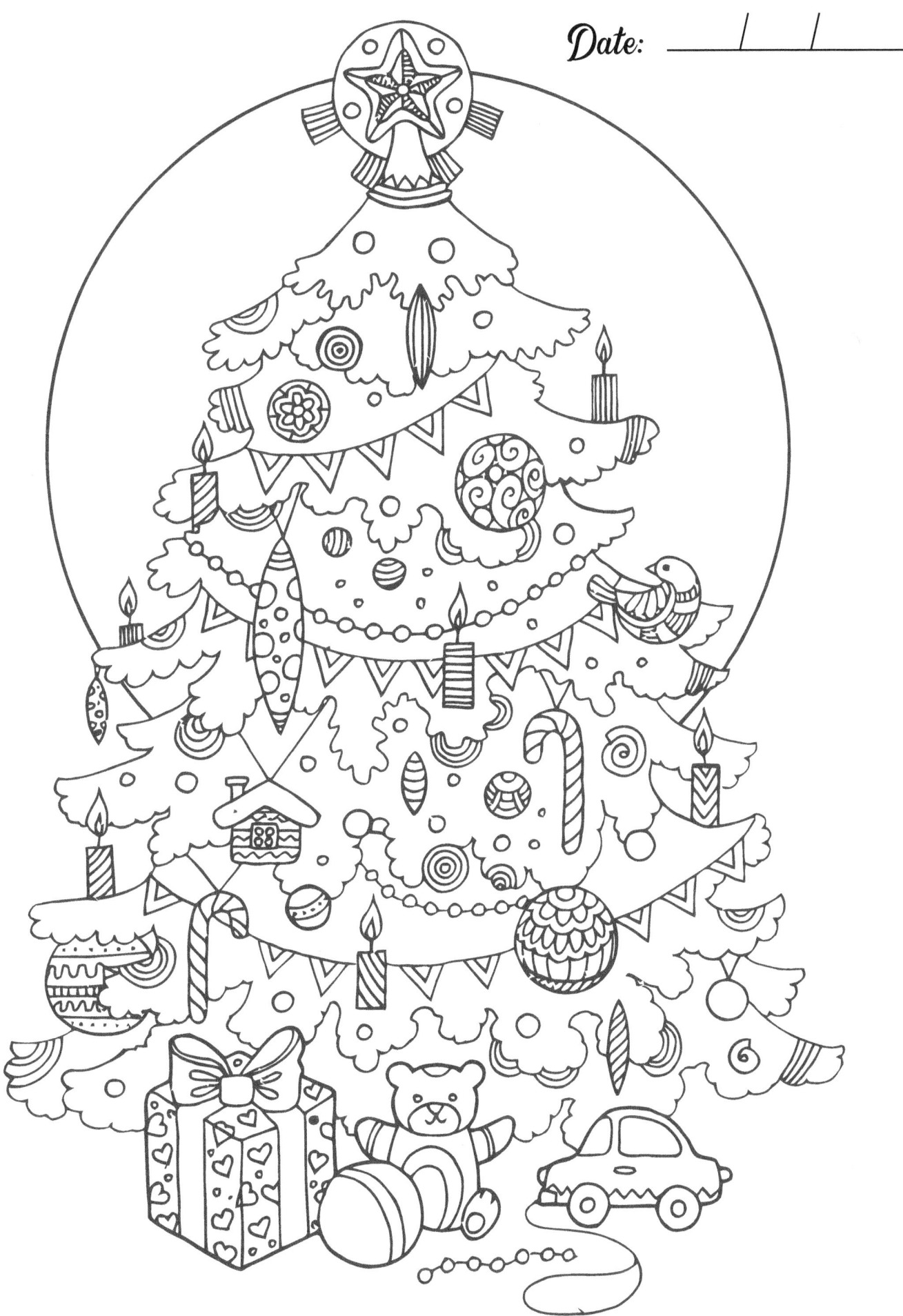

Write and Draw to Express Yourself

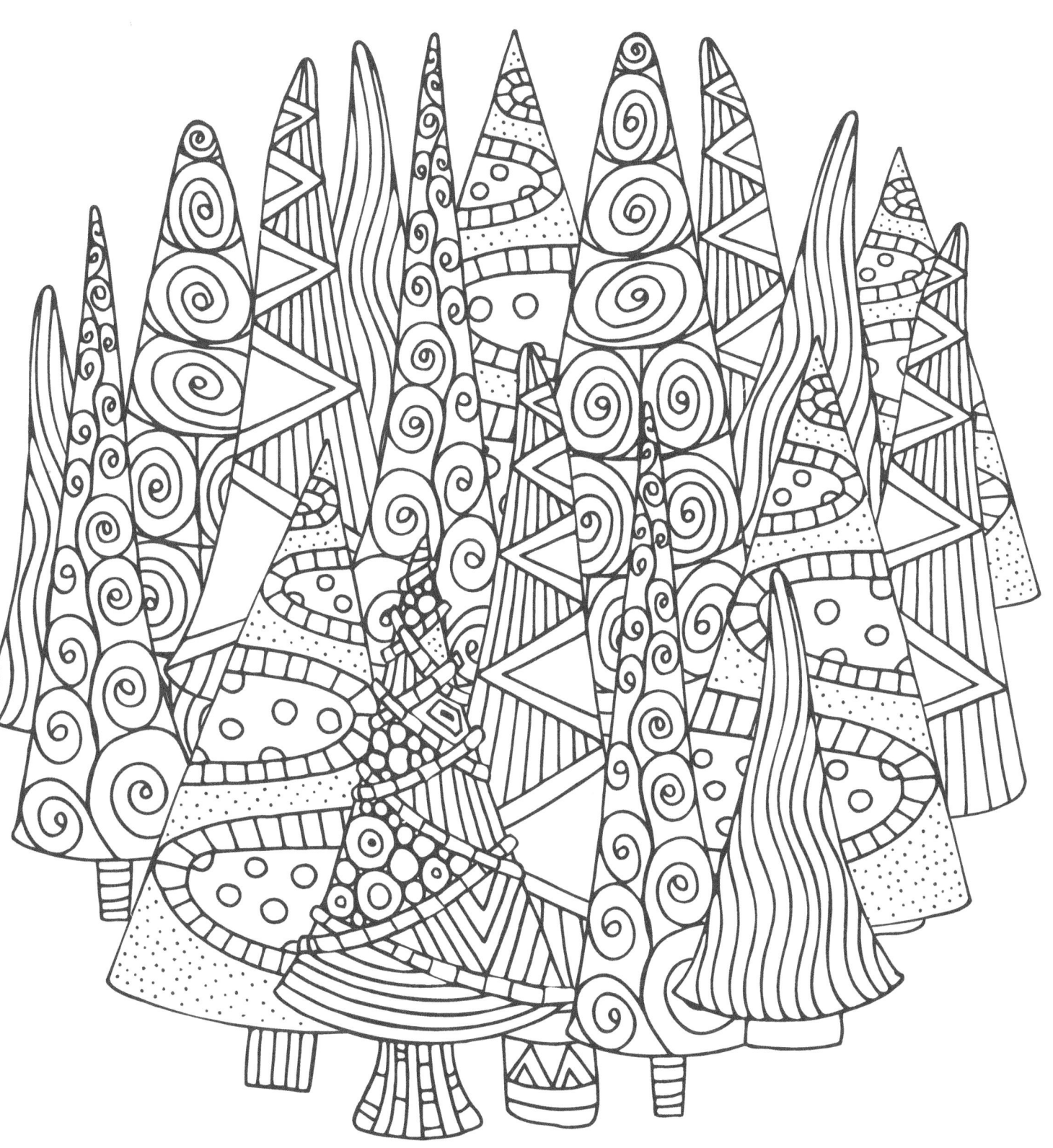

Write and Draw to Express Yourself

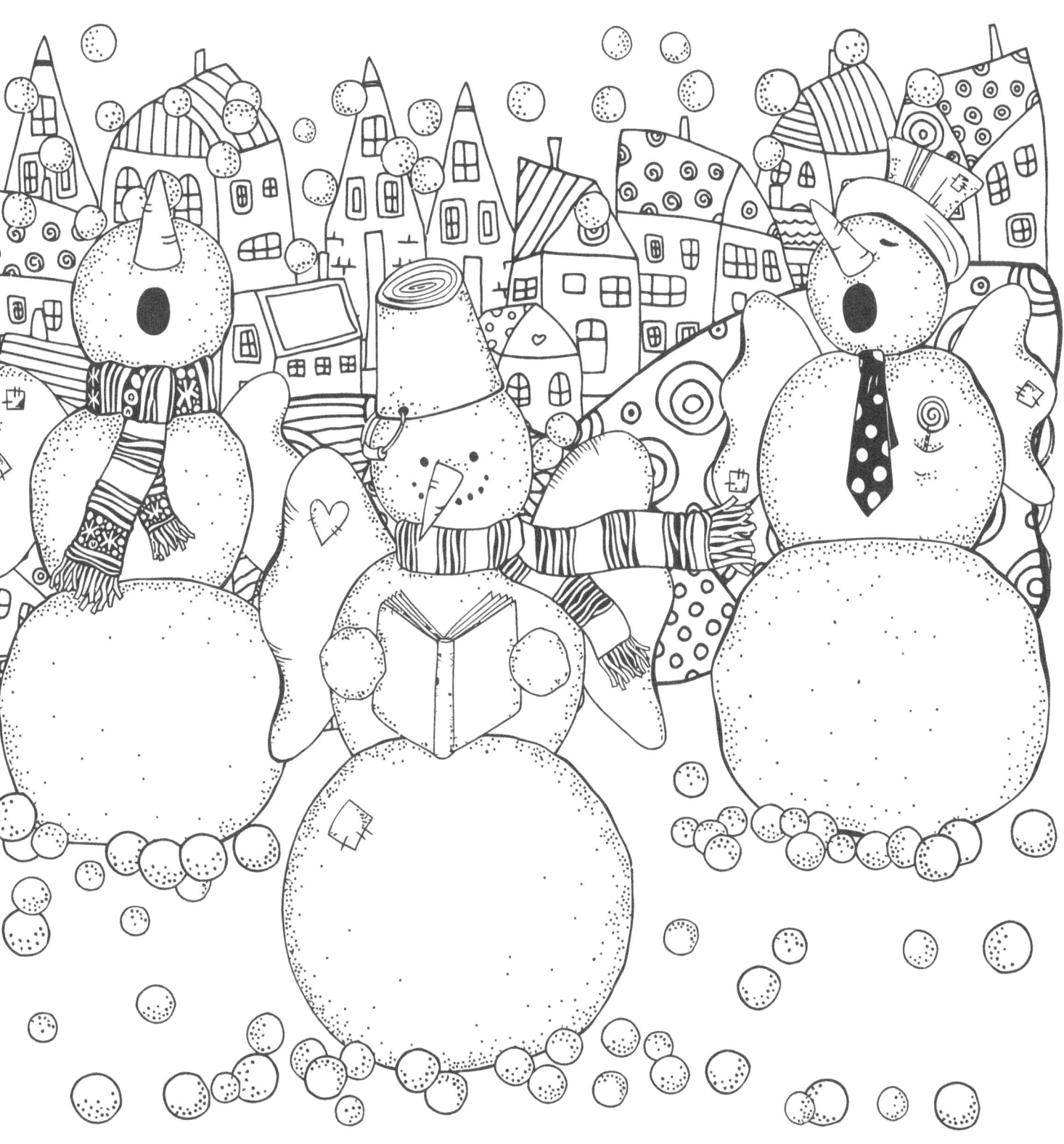

Write and Draw to Express Yourself

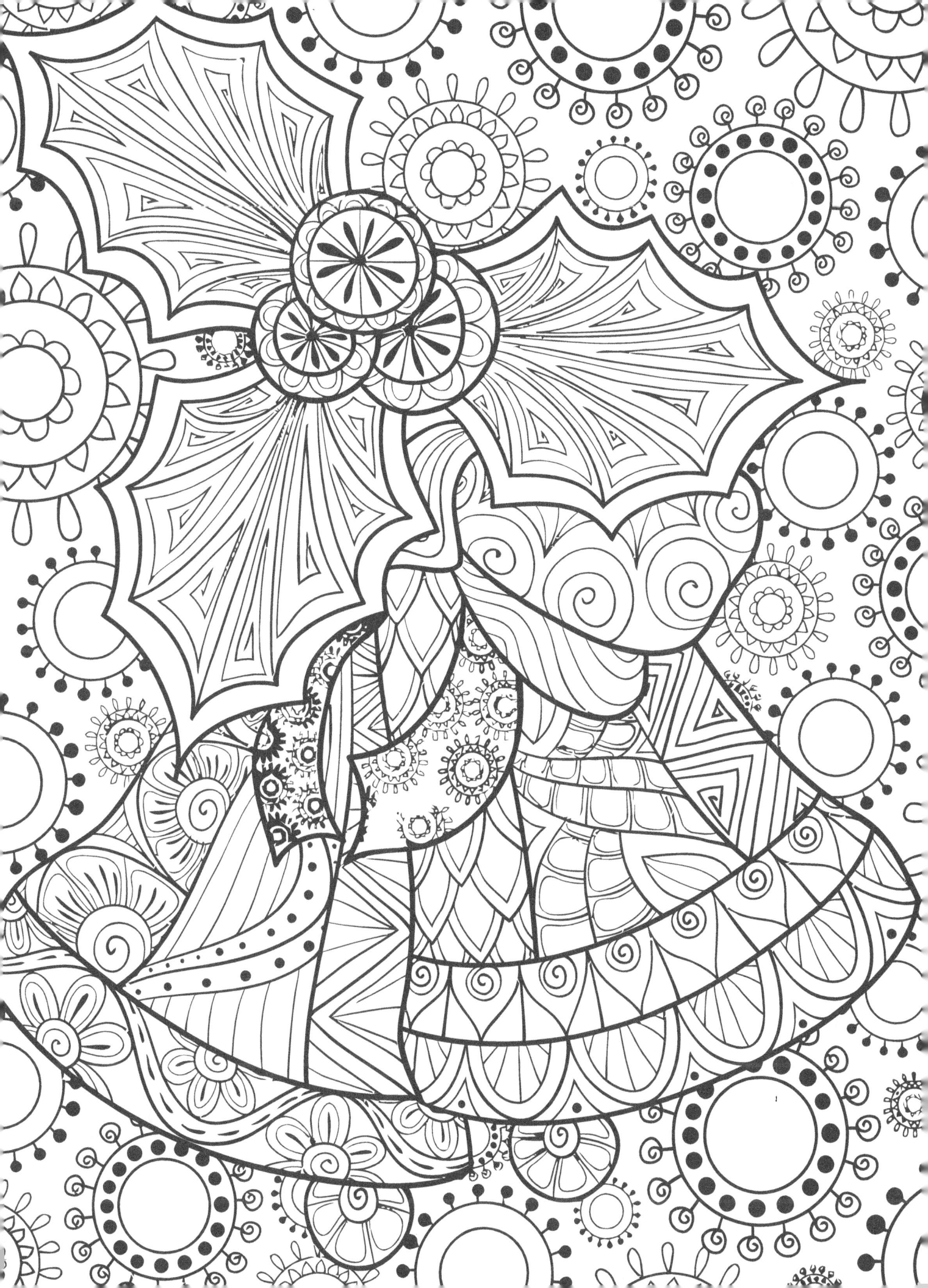

Write and Draw to Express Yourself

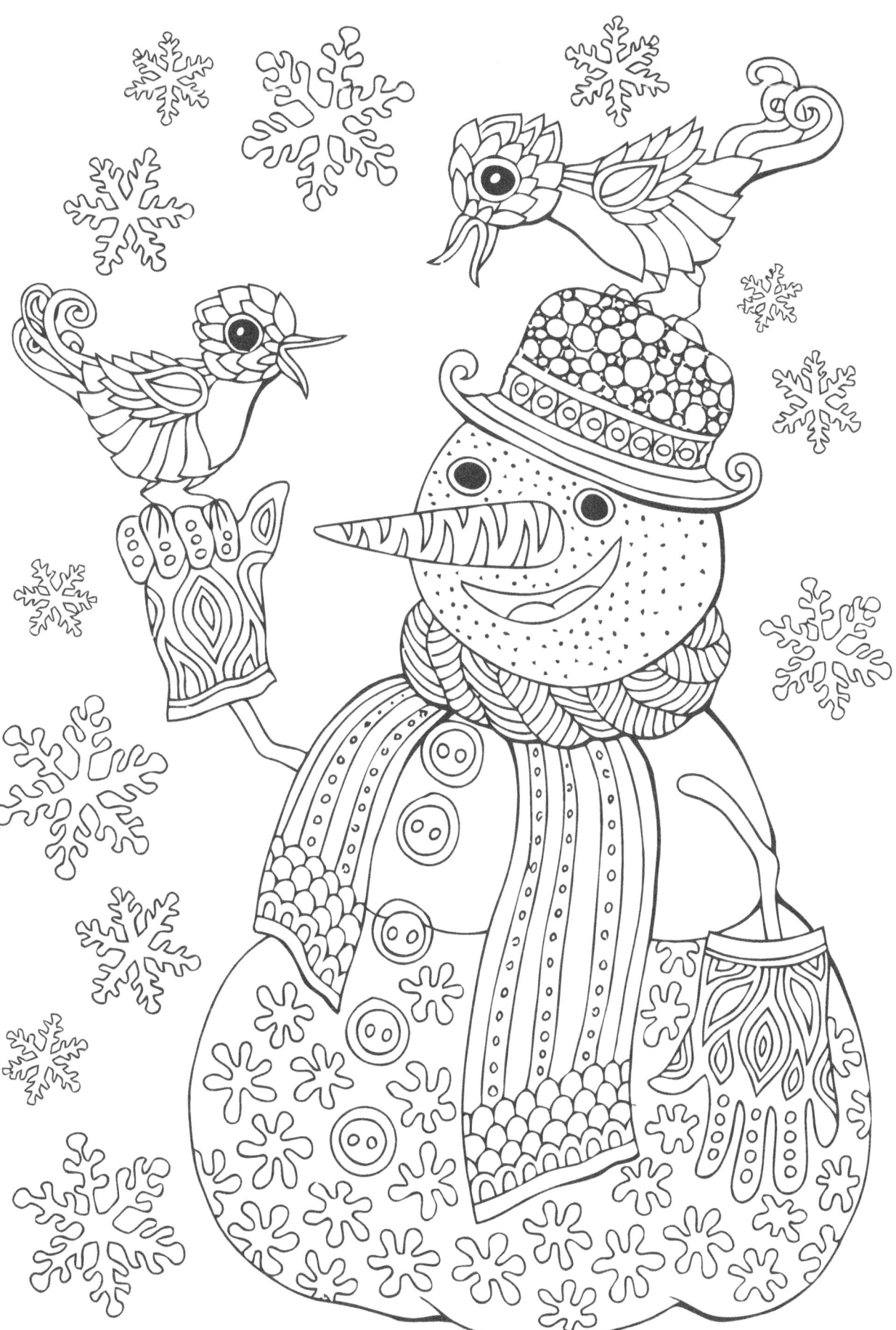

Write and Draw to Express Yourself

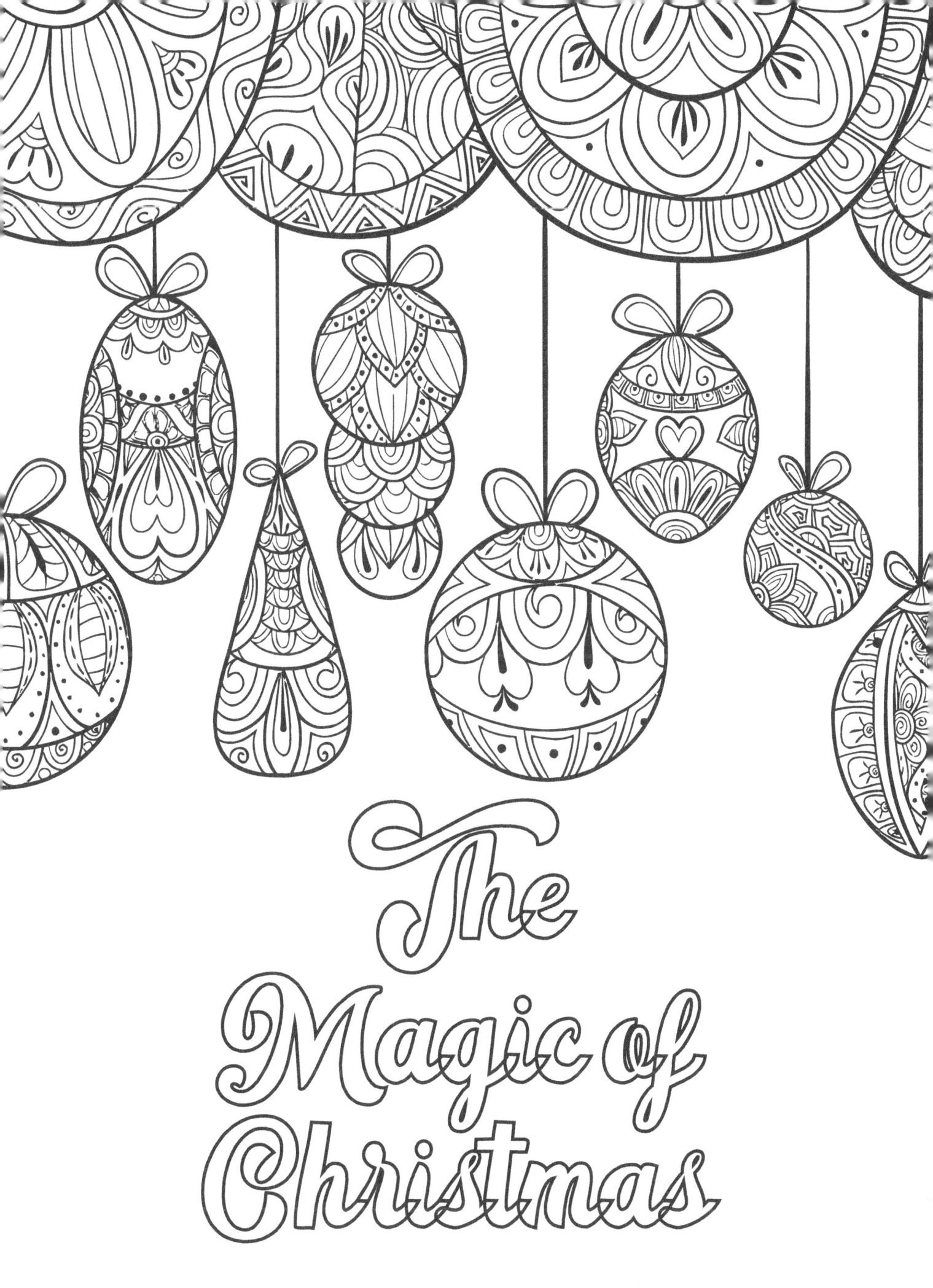

Write and Draw to Express Yourself

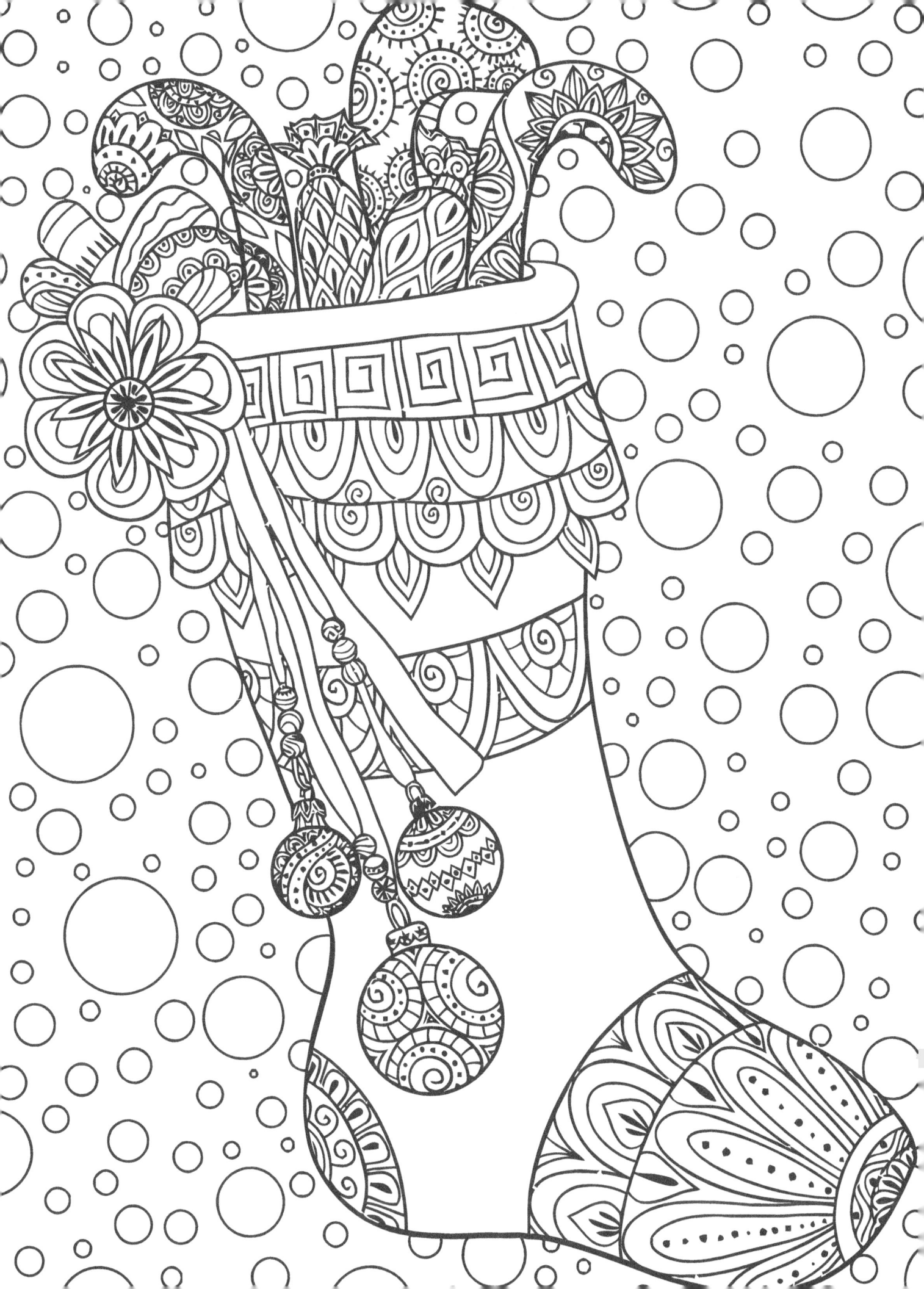

Write and Draw to Express Yourself

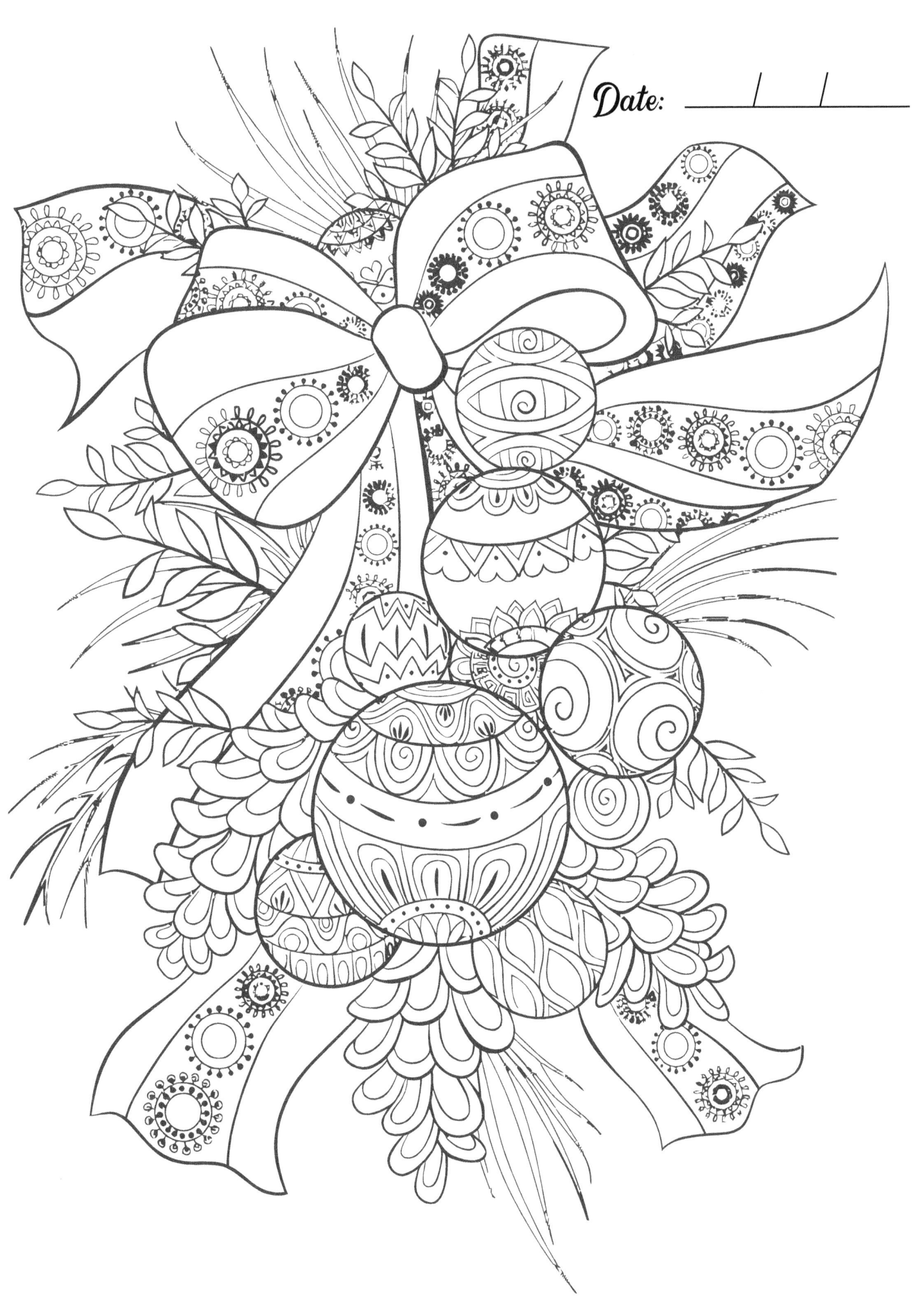

Write and Draw to Express Yourself

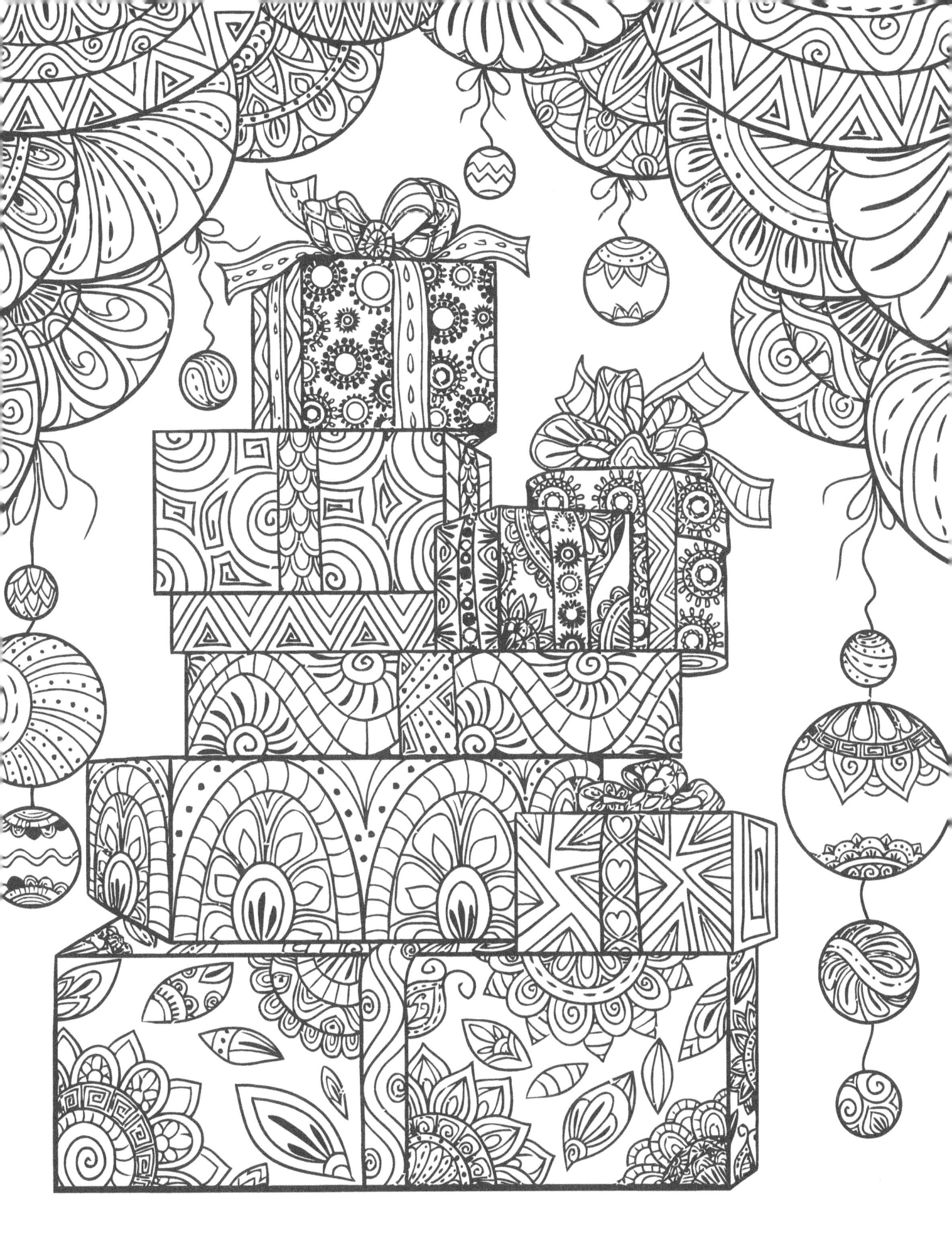

Write and Draw to Express Yourself

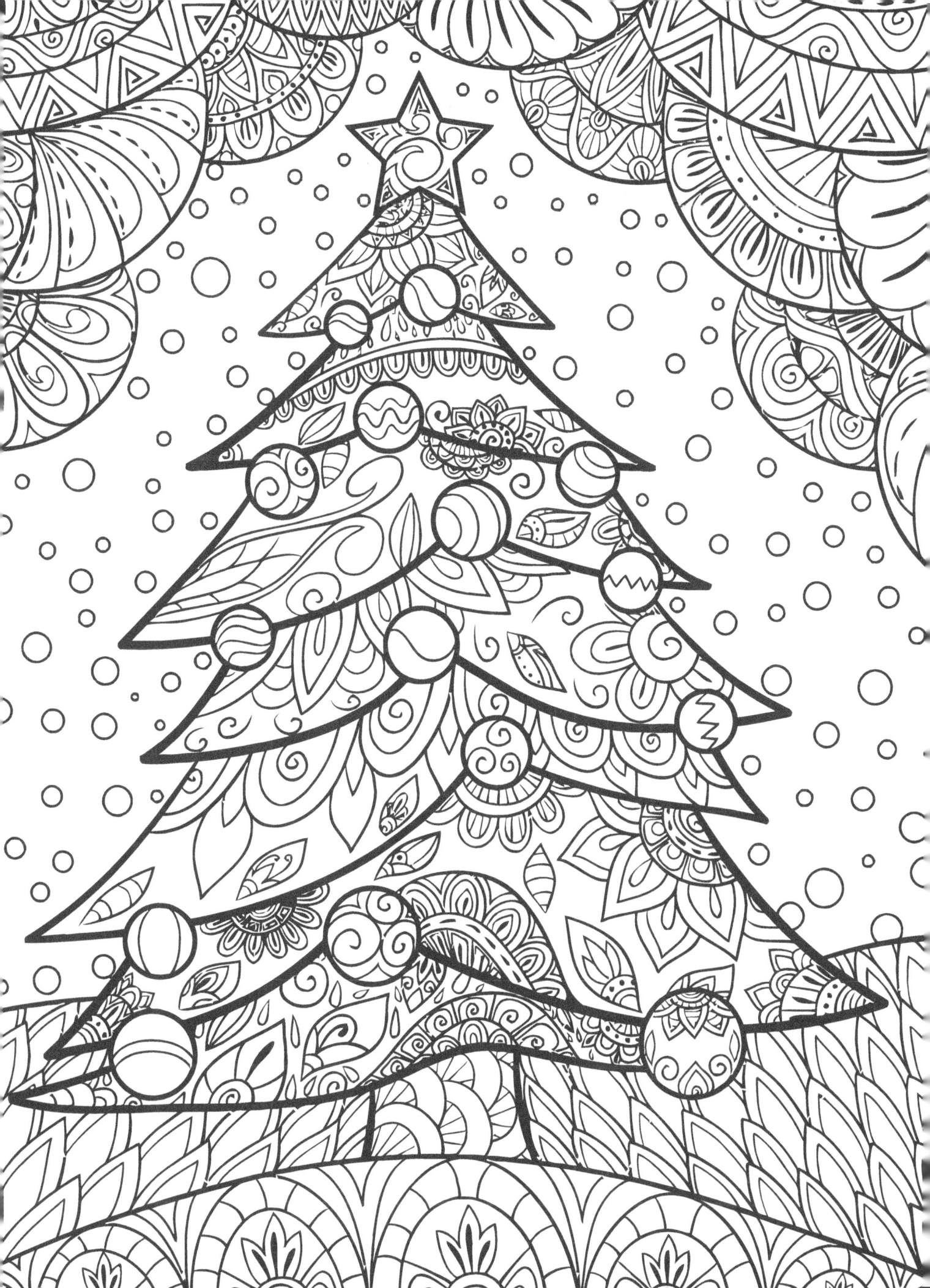

Write and Draw to Express Yourself

Date: _____ / ___ / ___

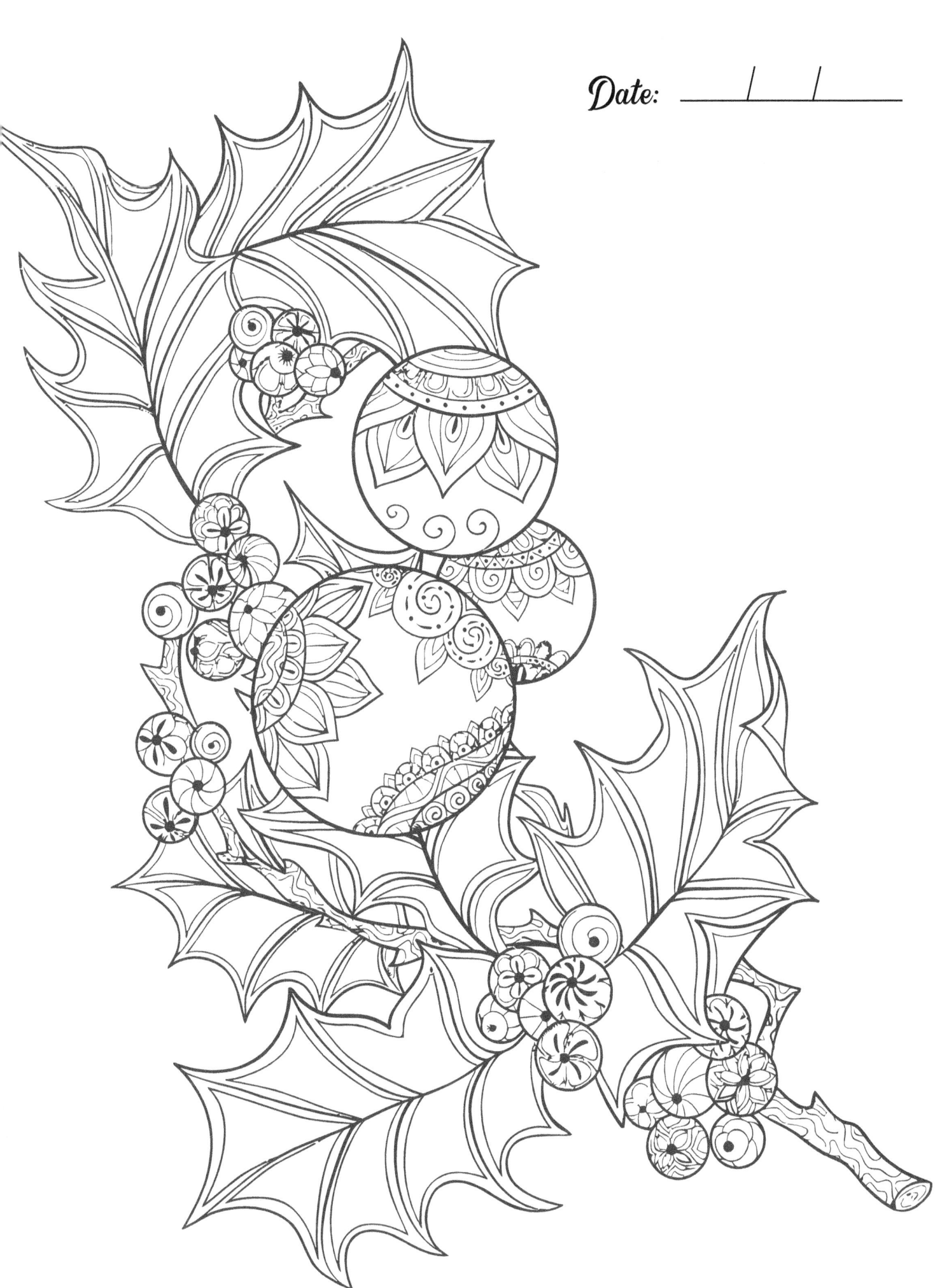

Write and Draw to Express Yourself

Date: _____ / ____ / ____

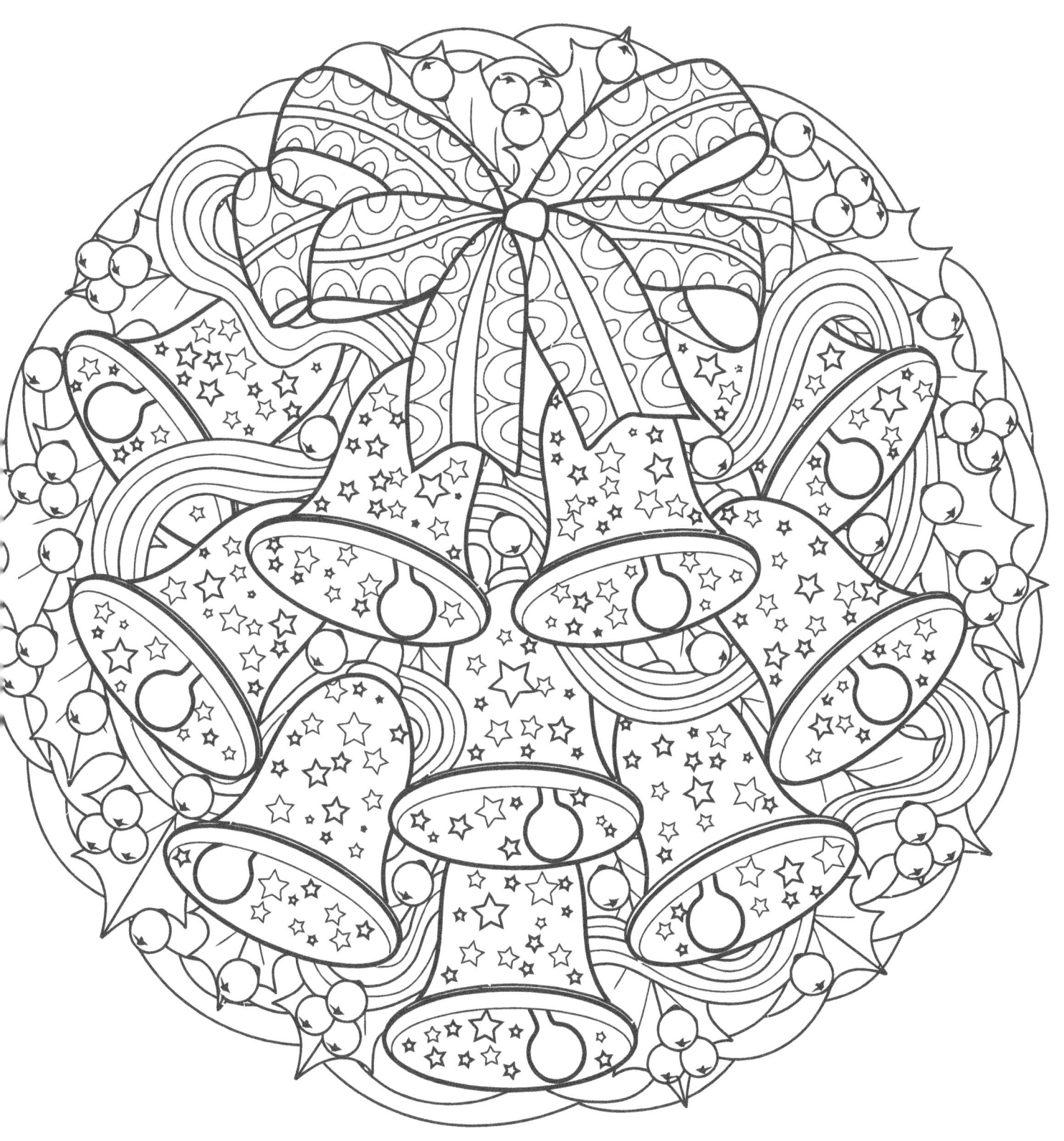

Write and Draw to Express Yourself

Write and Draw to Express Yourself

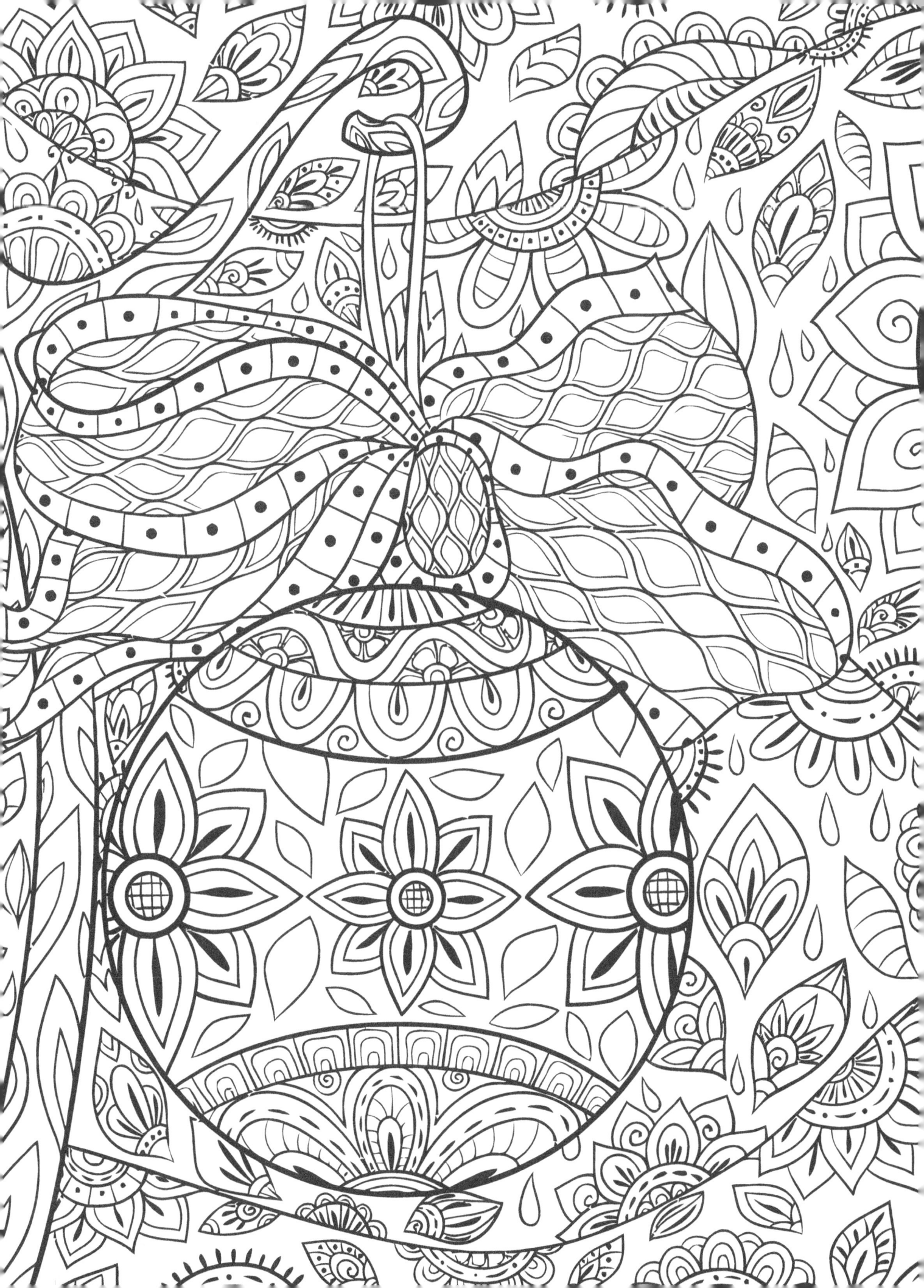

Write and Draw to Express Yourself

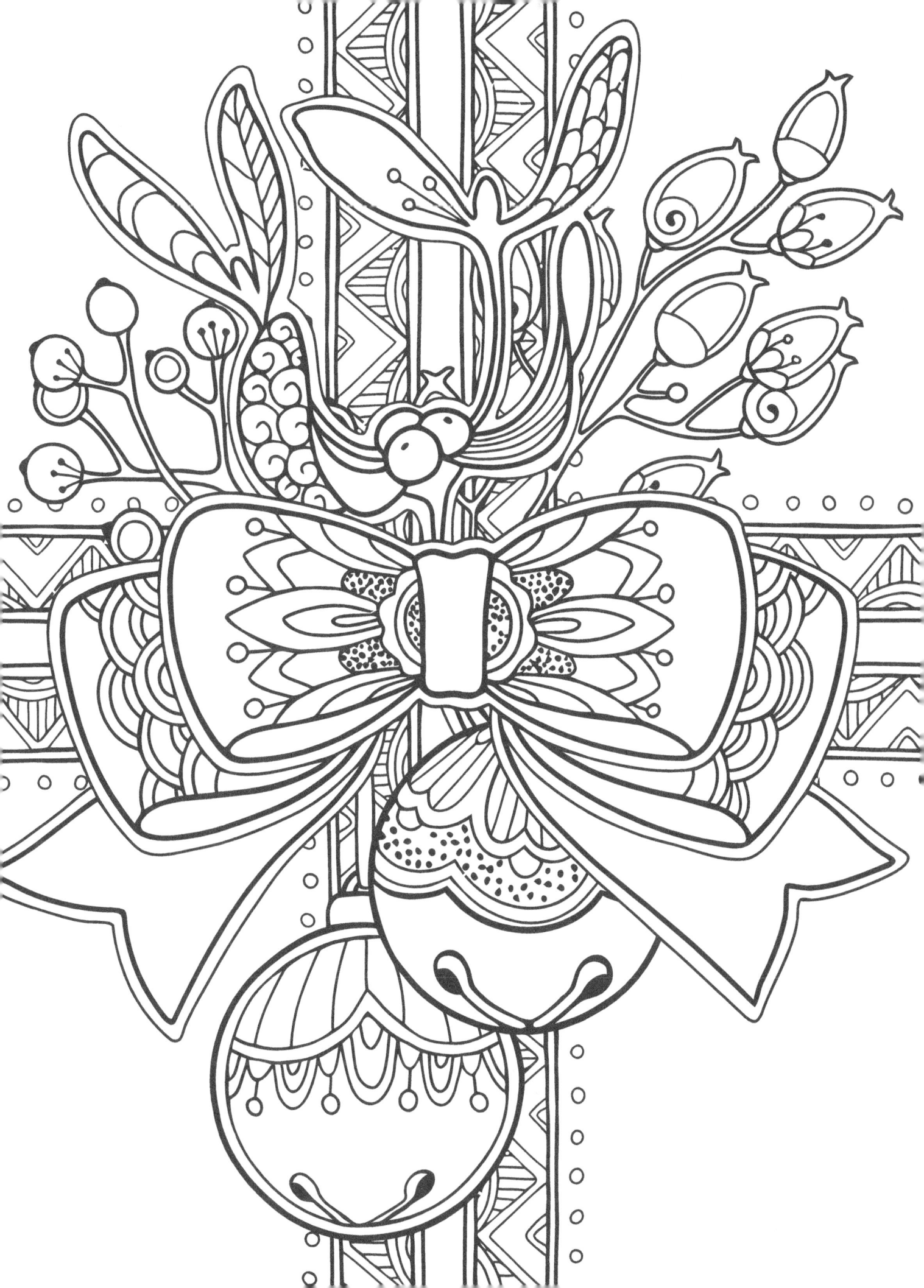

Write and Draw to Express Yourself

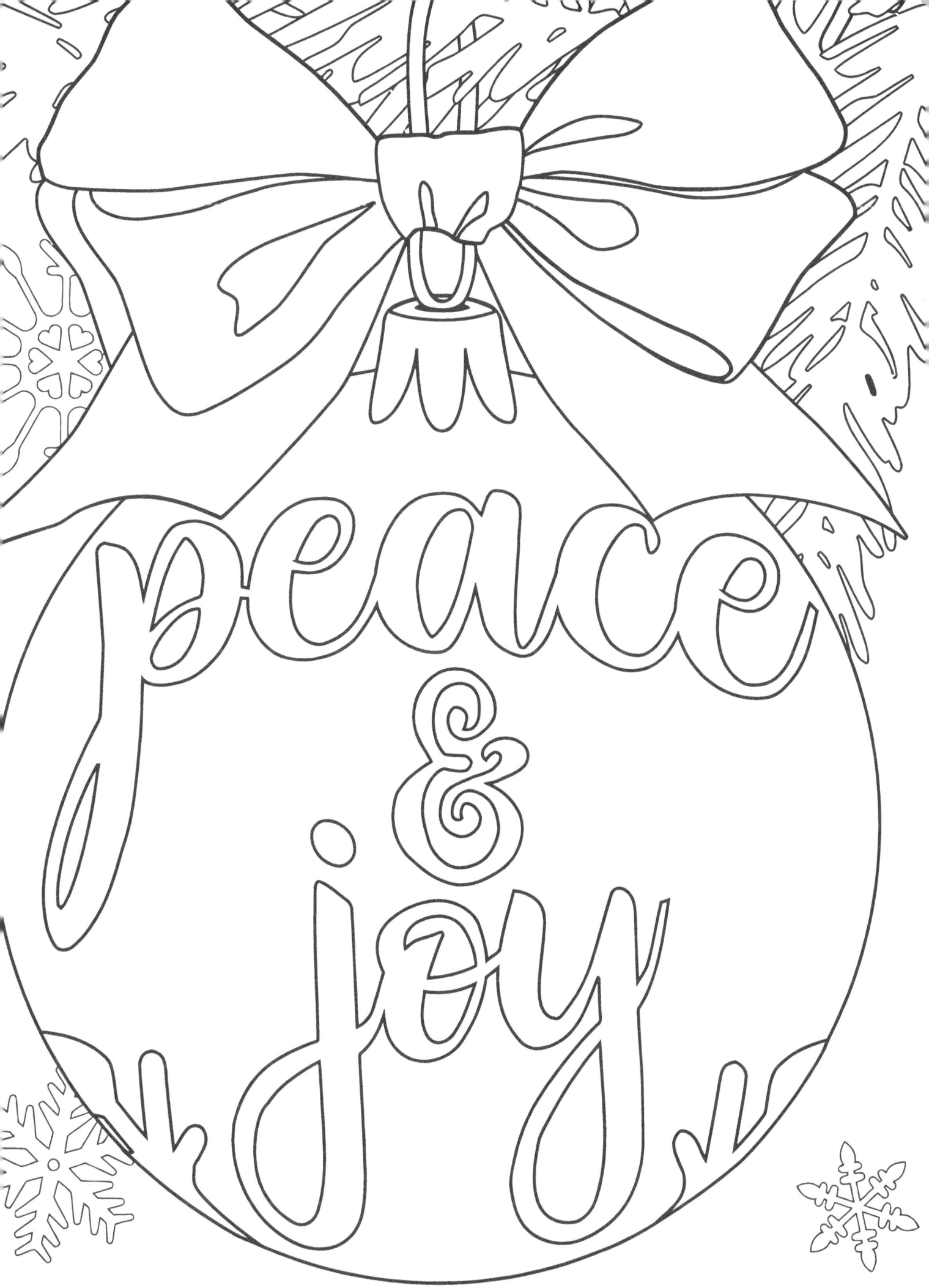

Write and Draw to Express Yourself

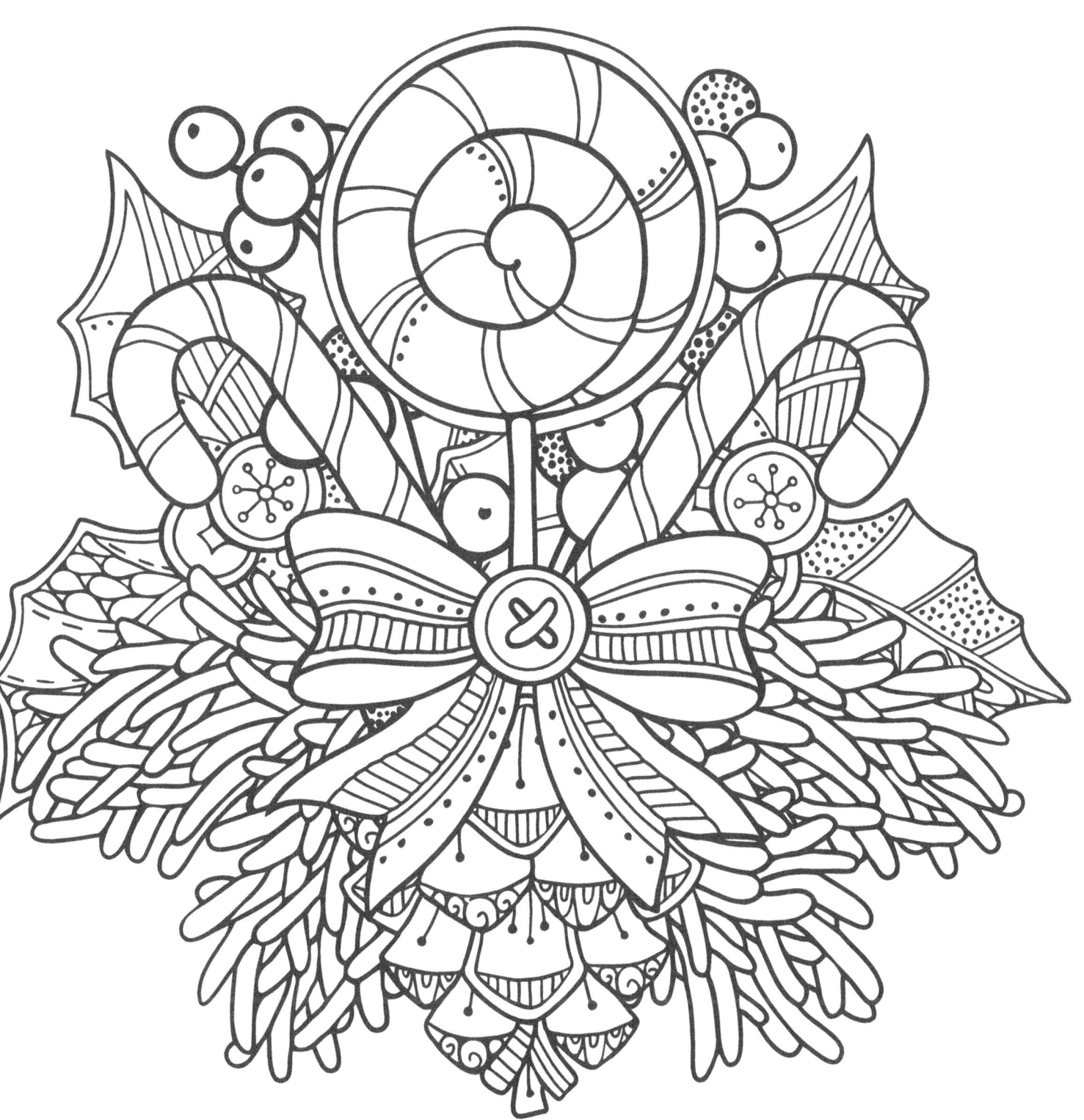

Write and Draw to Express Yourself

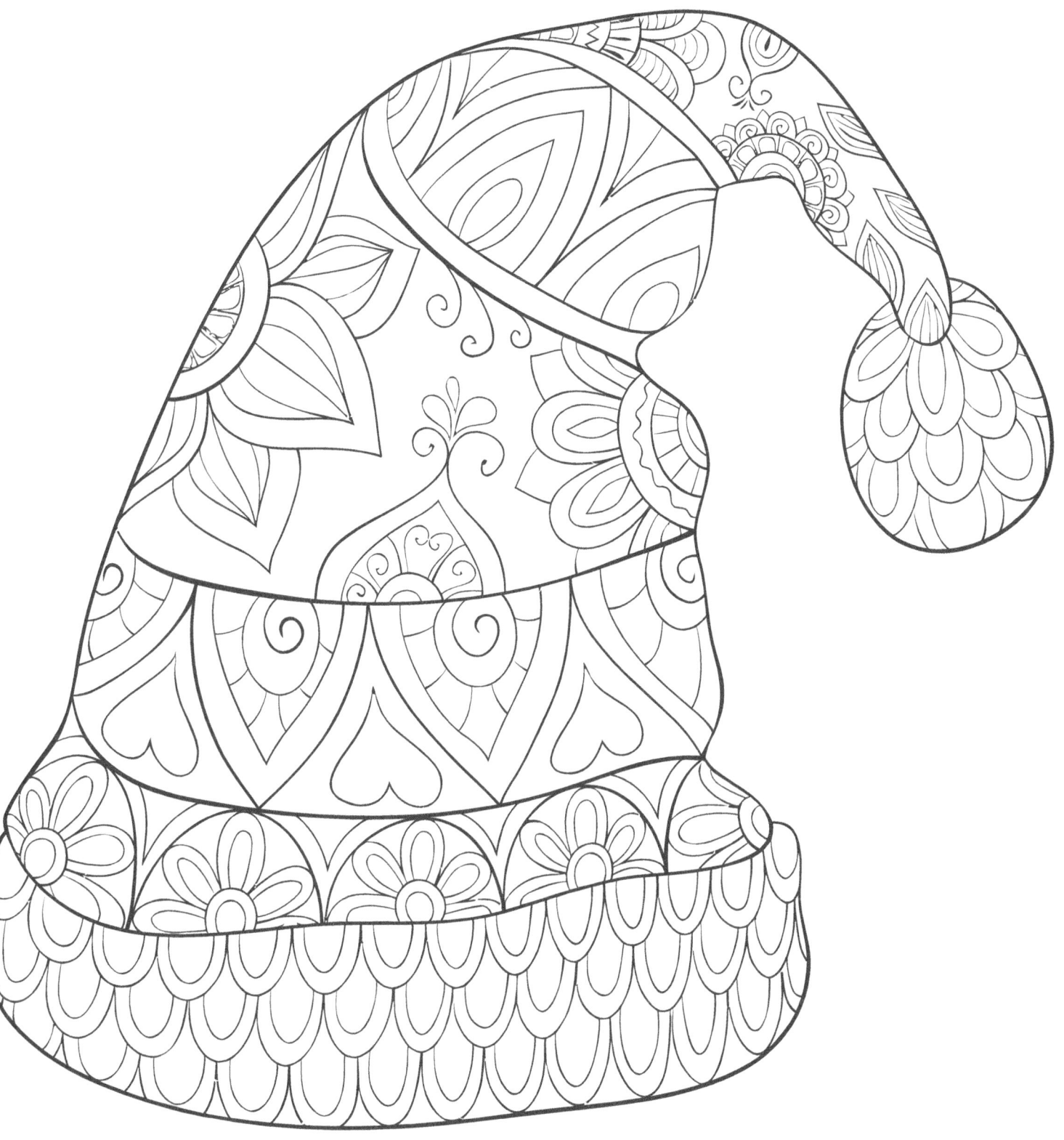

Write and Draw to Express Yourself

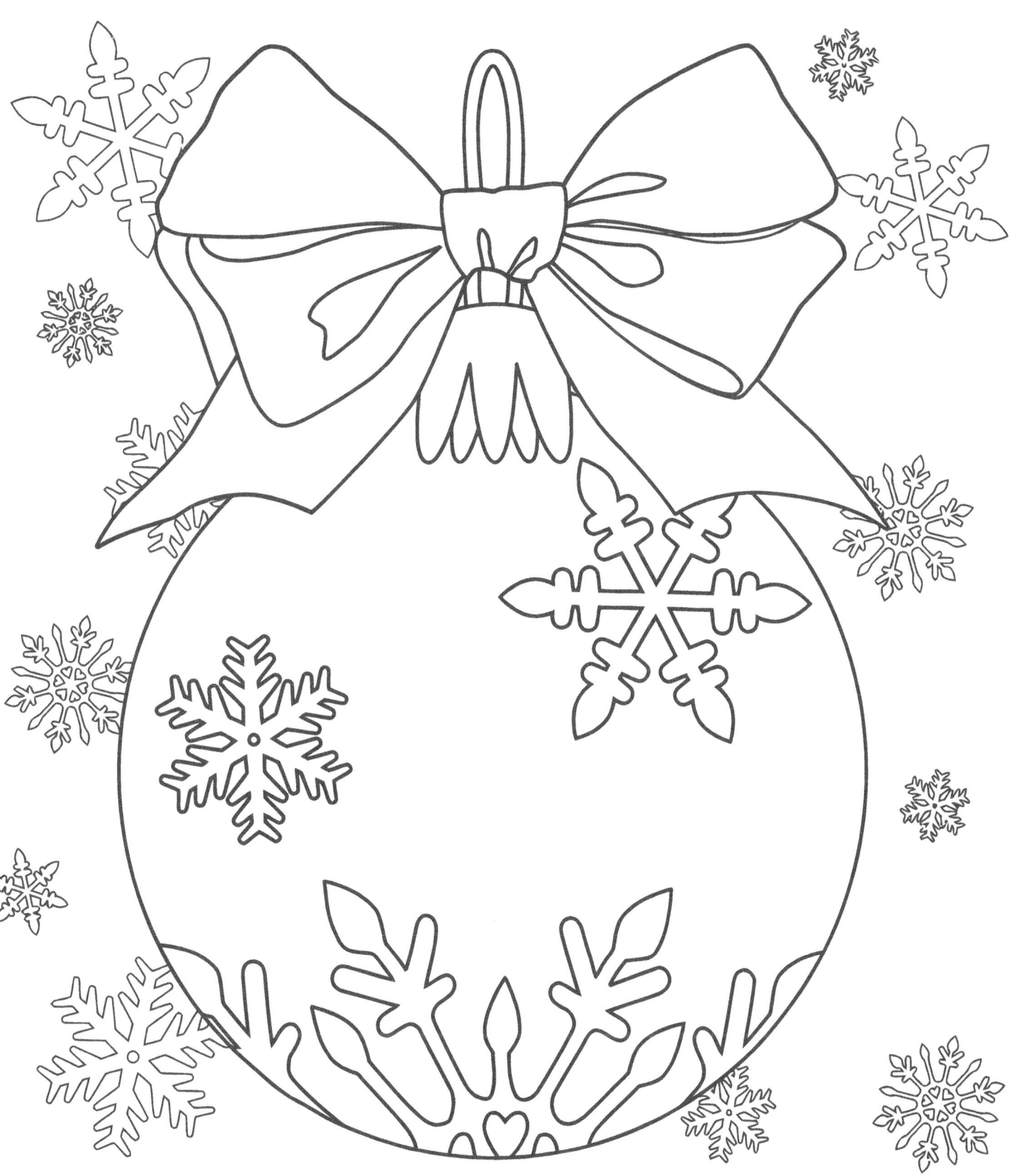

Write and Draw to Express Yourself

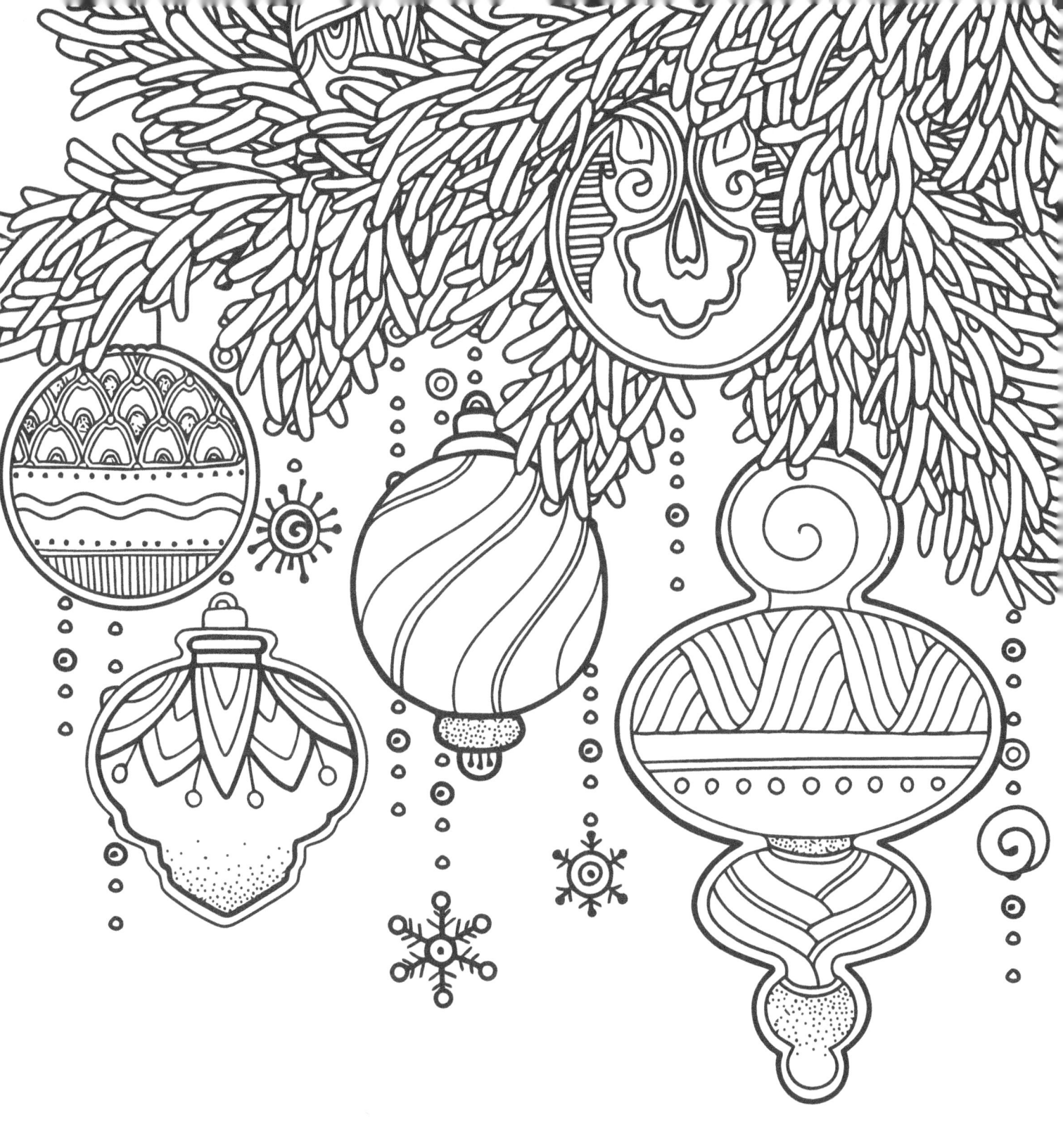

Write and Draw to Express Yourself

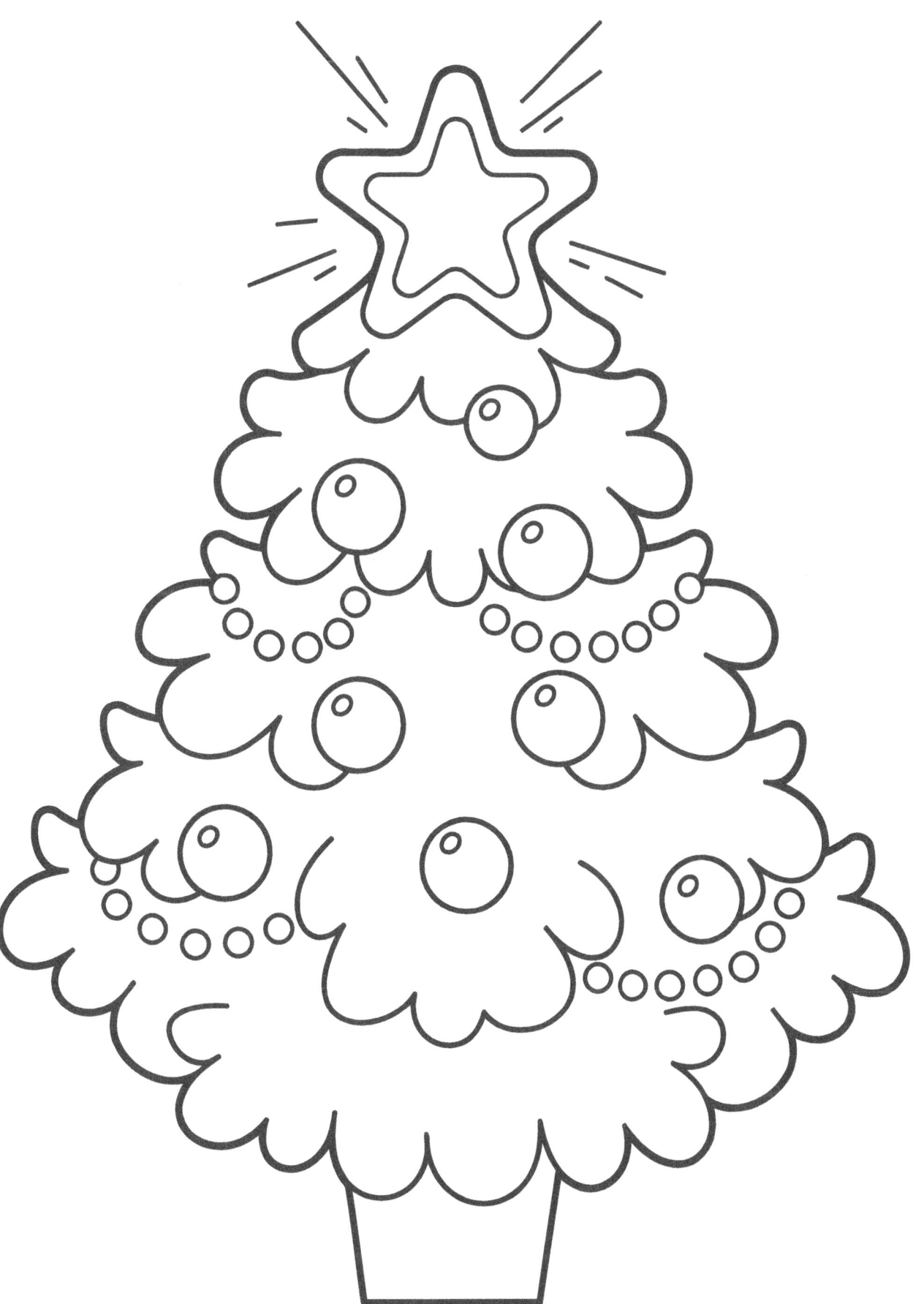

Write and Draw to Express Yourself

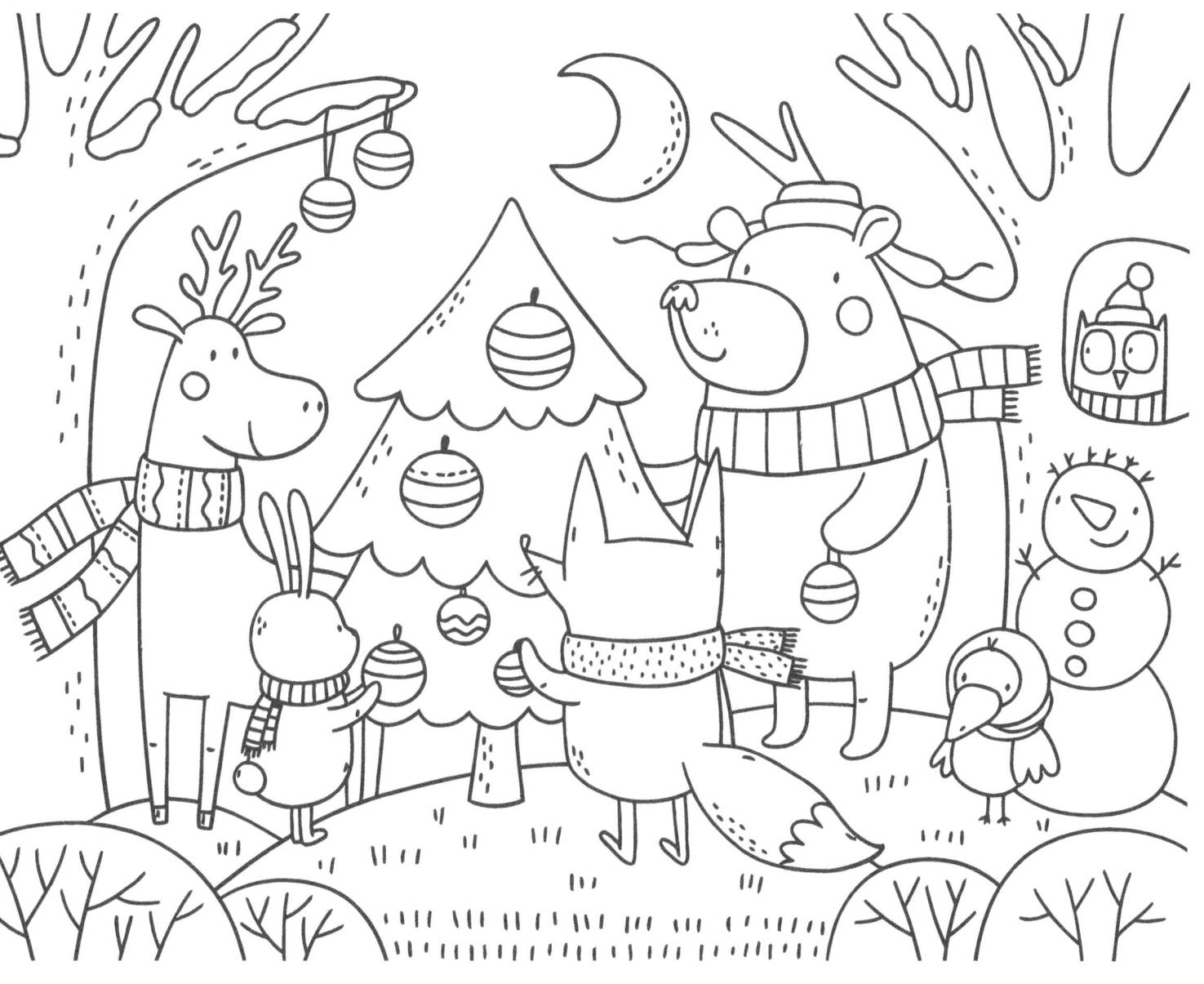

Write and Draw to Express Yourself

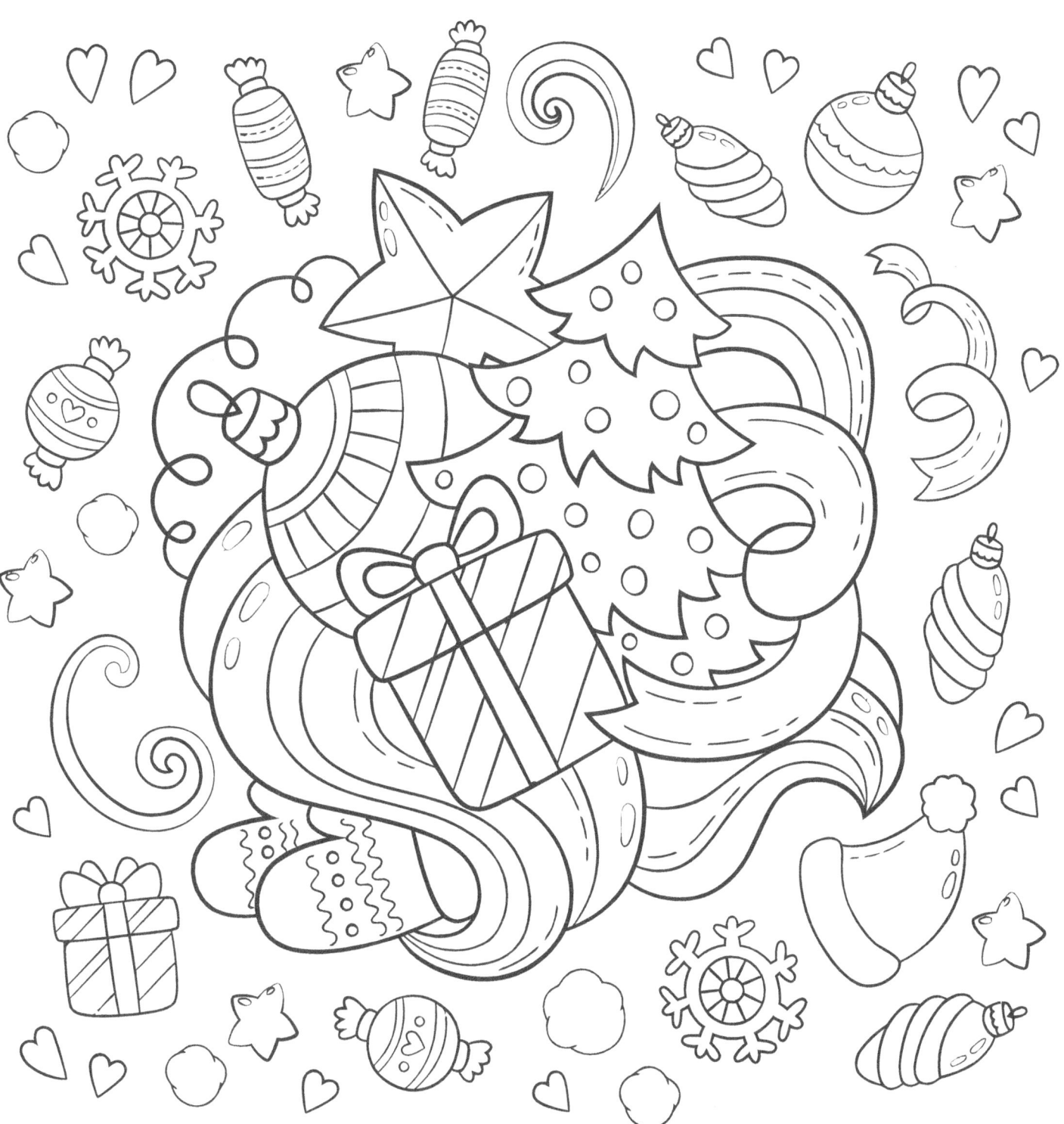

Write and Draw to Express Yourself

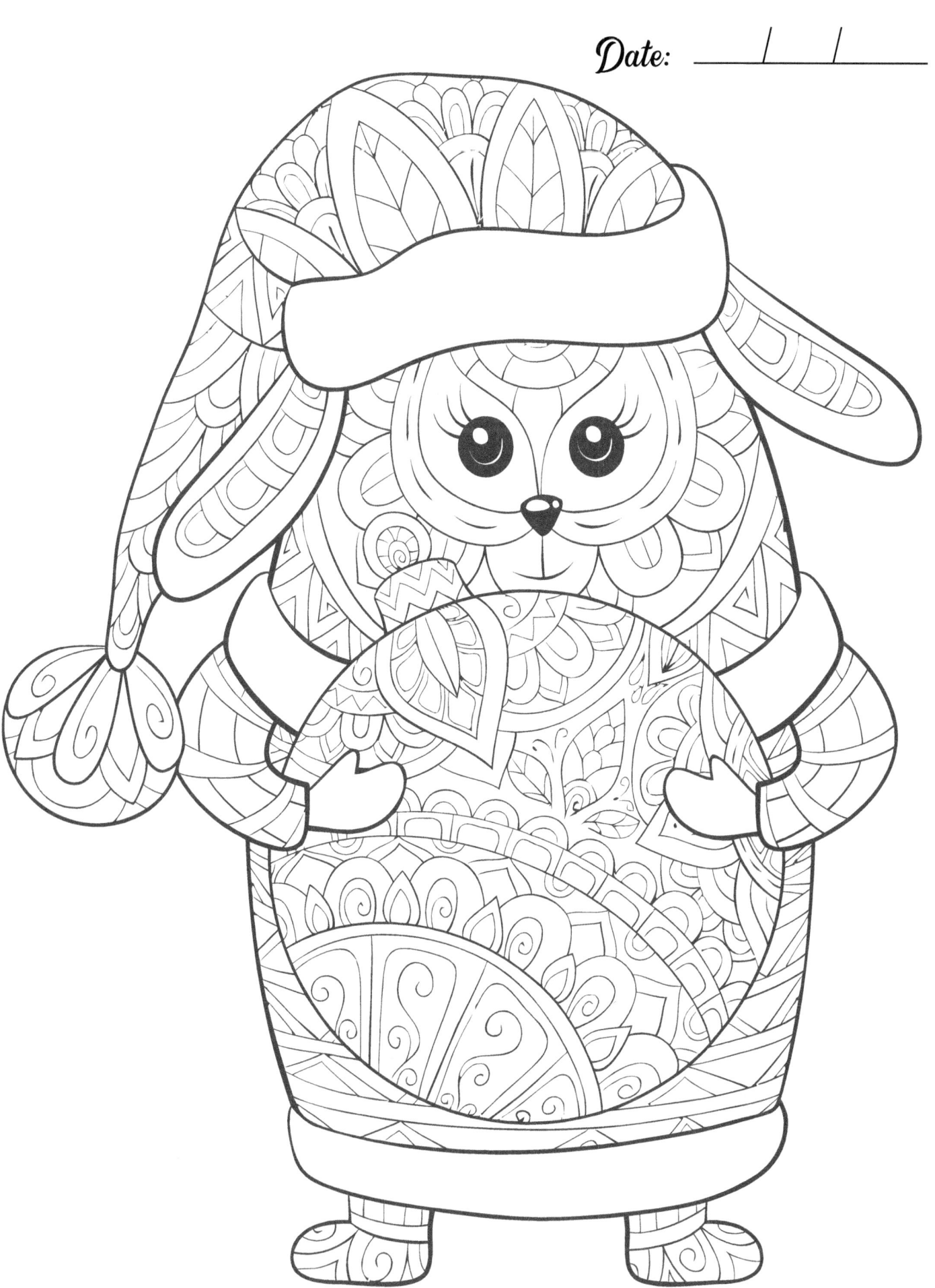

www.ingramcontent.com/pod-product-compliance
Lightning Source LLC
Chambersburg PA
CBHW081532220526
45467CB00010B/3151